The Tongue
An Evil Master...A Good Servant

Let the words of my mouth, and the meditation of my heart, be acceptable in thy sight, O Lord, my strength, and my redeemer. Psalm 19:14

By Ivet Graham-Morgan

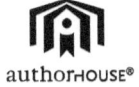
authorHOUSE®

AuthorHouse™
1663 Liberty Drive, Suite 200
Bloomington, IN 47403
www.authorhouse.com
Phone: 1-800-839-8640

First published by AuthorHouse 5/19/2008

ISBN: 978-1-4343-7096-9 (sc)

Library of Congress Control Number: 2008903485

Printed in the United States of America
Bloomington, Indiana

This book is printed on acid-free paper.

Dedication

To mankind everywhere

Table of Contents

Preface

I wrote this book with the intent of encouraging others; believers and unbelievers alike, to submit themselves completely to Jesus Christ and to obey His Word for only then can the tongue function in the fruit of the spirit rather than the works of the flesh. I am fully convinced that the tongue can only be tamed when our hearts seek to trade the works of the flesh for the fruit of the spirit. The character of Satan resides in every life that is not God-centered and therefore such individuals become potential candidates to be used in the works of the flesh.

The existence of Satan should not be trivialized; we must understand that Satan is a real enemy and spiritual warfare is going on all around us—whether we're aware of it or not. Satan is as real as the air we breathe and so we must never allow ourselves to be convinced that Satan does not exist. Satan is an enemy and a master at camouflaging and marketing himself in attractive packages. Jesus knows Satan is a powerful adversary for He was there when Satan fell like lightning from heaven as documented in **Luke**

10:18. Jesus has made it clear that Satan has authority on earth as both the (self-proclaimed) ruler and prince of this world **John 12:31, 14:30, and 16:11.**

During His time on this earth Jesus spent much time in prayer—an example for us as adherents to do likewise. It is only when we stay in ceaseless communication with God, allowing the spirit dominance over the flesh, that we can discern the sneaky plans of the enemy layered in what appears to be desirable wrappers. Jesus was able to recognize Satan hiding in Peter and quickly rebuked him. There are many who yield to temptation through ignorance and then find themselves trapped by that crafty fox called Satan. We must spend time in prayer and fasting and in the Word of God so we will be equipped against the wiles of the devil. God states in his Word: **"My people are destroyed for lack of knowledge:"** (Hosea 4:6a) Always remember that the knowledge you require to live a spirit-filled life is readily available, directly to you, as you commune with your creator through prayer and through His Word as documented in the Holy Bible.

Over a five-year period, I have witnessed first hand how the sins of the tongue can completely alter the lives of those touched by it—careers ruined, reputations eradicated, marriages wrecked, families torn apart, suspicion breed, profound grief and pain accompanied by heartaches, headaches, nightmares, and considerable health deterioration. They were an average hard-working middle-class family until their world was turned upside down by malicious gossip and slander. As I watched the pain and suffering endured by the victims and their family members and observed their individual efforts to rebuild, I found myself focusing on the cancer that had annihilated this family rather than the perpetrators who had preyed upon them.

In my search for answers I turned to the Holy Bible, and after much searching and studying I concluded that Satan is a universal adversary of mankind who instigates, continuously, a myriad of evil ploys to bring suffering to mankind. Satan no longer has to depend on the serpent alone to carry out his diabolical schemes, for he now has a host of human beings on whom he can rely at a moment's notice.

The sins of the tongue are not confined to the secular world; in fact, they are quite rampant in the church today, even among those who have been ordained as officers of the gospel of Jesus Christ. I was away from home for almost a year, starting in the fall of 2005 to the early summer of 2006. During this period, I worshipped at a church where on several occasions I observed believers who identified themselves as 'born again Christians' openly engaging in the sins of the tongue. On one occasion after the morning services, I was in the basement area where snacks and lunches are available. While there, an elderly sister walked in, she was in tears. When concerned members of the group asked what was wrong, she named a certain deaconess and between sobs she briefly divulged that this deaconess had told lies about her. She was comforted and encouraged by others and although she appeared calm for a while, one could tell she was still hurting and finally she went home for the day. Being a visitor, I did not know the deaconess she had named but a few weeks later I met this deaconess—I realized right away that her face was familiar even though I could not associate the face with a name.

Once again we were in the basement area of the church after the morning service. We were having lunch and this particular deaconess joined the group at the table— I learned her name then. While eating, she voiced her displeasure concerning a rule that had been put into effect regarding the placement of children during the Sunday morning worship service. As she voiced her disapproval at the table everyone listened but no one commented. Later, during the evening services, at the time of the announcements, the pastor mentioned this particular deaconess by name stating that she had brought it to his attention that some believers were complaining about the foolishness of 'Children's Church' as they felt the children should not be sent off to their own service but should be allowed to participate in the general adult service. The minister invited those who had concerns to voice them to him and not to attack him in quiet. He took a quick poll of those with children and then threw out the invitation for those with concerns to voice them. Overwhelmingly, the church applauded 'Children's Church' citing the many advantages that went along with it—there was not one person that disagreed with having the children accommodated in this fashion. They all saw this as a good arrangement where children could be reached at their own level and also they saw it as a way of avoiding the many disruptions that come from children when the minister is preaching.

I was astounded when the minister mentioned that this particular officer had brought it to his attention that others were complaining when in fact she was the only complainer at the table. She did all the talking while everyone else concentrated on eating; no one offered a comment to refute or to affirm her claim. To an unbeliever, this deaconess could very well become a stumbling block—using the same tongue to praise God and to lie with intent to slander. Her ungodly action could very well have caused irreparable damage within the church had the pastor not handled the situation the way he did. This particular officer was very visible in the church—having her seat in the front row on the podium with other officers of the gospel and carried out many important functions. She was actively involved in church duties, among these, the serving of the Lord's Supper. Unfortunately, during my brief stay at this church she was not the only officer involved in various sins of the tongue—inwardly, I questioned the sincerity of these people as followers of Christ. The reality of using Christ as one's example, rather than man, also came forcefully home to me. James puts this kind of behaviour into perspective when he said:

> **"Therewith bless we God, even the Father; and therewith curse we men, which are made after the similitude of God. Out of the same mouth proceedeth blessing and cursing. My brethren, these things ought not so to be. Doth a fountain send forth at the same place sweet water and bitter? Can the fig tree, my brethren, bear olive berries? either a vine, figs? so can no fountain both yield salt water and fresh."** (James 3:9-12)

This type of conduct in the Christian community is rather unacceptable on all levels—sin and righteousness can never be wrapped in the same cloak. Our commitment to Christ has to be 100 percent or nothing—the 'half-and-half' theory just won't work when it comes to serving and worshipping God. In Matthew 6:24 Jesus made it clear, **"No man can serve two masters: for either he will hate the one, and love the other; or else he will hold to the** one, and despise the other. **You cannot serve God and mammom."**

I have since discovered that in many churches nowadays, the sins of the tongue have somehow become amenable and commonplace. Sins of the tongue such as gossiping, backbiting, and slandering are viewed as little mischievous practices that are not really so serious—they belong to the minor league. This is, without doubt, another lie coated in deceit straight from the pit of hell. In Romans 1:28-32 Paul made it clear in his letter to the church in Rome that such sins are in the same league as murder, sexual sins, and a host of other horrendous acts and that those who commit them are worthy of death.

In Matthew Chapter 4:1-11, Jesus had a personal experienced with Satan during His forty days in the wilderness when He faced real temptations from Satan. Knowing that Satan would come after us as well, Jesus has taught us to pray: **"Our Father which art in heaven, Hallowed be thy name...And lead us not into temptation but deliver us from evil..."** (Matthew 6:6-13) Jesus also prayed personally for our protection in the prayer documented in John 17.

Jesus also warned about Satan's interference in our lives. He taught in one parable documented in Matthew 13:24-30 that the kingdom of heaven is like a man who sowed good seed in his field. But while everyone was sleeping, his enemy came and sowed tares (a problematic weed) among the wheat, and went away.

The tares in this parable represent the agents of the devil and the enemy who sows the tares is the devil. The enemy came unnoticed because everyone was asleep—that is exactly how Satan operates even today and that is why Paul warns us to put on the whole armor of God. The sins of the tongue have a way of slipping in silently and sneakily.

Purpose within your heart that you will not be a casualty of Satan; make your walk with Christ a close one, beginning now—*only Christ is your example, keep your eyes on Him and **not** on man.*

All scriptures quoted throughout this book are taken from the King James Version.

Ivet Graham-Morgan
Ontario, Canada
February 20, 2008

"Only let your conversation be as it becometh the gospel of Christ: that whether I come and see you, or else be absent, I may hear of your affairs, that ye stand fast in one spirit, with one mind striving together for the faith of the gospel;"

(Philippians 1:27)

Man The Created Being

"God is a Spirit: and they that worship Him
must worship Him in Spirit and in truth"
(John 4:24)

To truly understand the reason the tongue of mankind cannot be tamed except through submission to God we have to take a look at man in the Garden of Eden before the fall, and the relationship he had with his creator then. The Bible says, **"And God said, Let us make man in our image, after our likeness: and let them have dominion over the fish of the sea, and over the fowl of the air, and over the cattle, and over all the earth, and over every creeping thing that creepeth upon the earth."** (Genesis 1:26) **"And the Lord God formed man of the dust of the ground, and breathed into his nostrils the breath of life; and man became a living soul."** (Genesis 2:7)

The first man was not only created perfect, he also had a personal relationship with his Creator and was in harmony with himself and with the world around him.

God placed him in the garden with his wife. There, they would live and care for the garden. They had dominion over God's creation and constant communication with God—work was not a burden but rather the relationship of mankind with God in maintaining the visible creation. Unimpaired, the first man was disciplined in his whole being and was free from the powerful feelings of physical desire that subdued him to the pleasures of the senses—self-centredness and covetousness for earthly goods, contrary to the order of rationale. When Adam and Eve opened the door to desire they gave admission to every lust of the flesh; and with this, sinfulness blemished their descendants—all of humanity. Thus, they changed the course of mankind. We read in 1 Corinthians 15:21-22: **"For since by man came death, by man came also the resurrection of the dead. For as in Adam all die, even so in Christ shall all be made alive."**

Man is a composition of a material element and a spiritual element, each needs the other to complement the whole—the human being. While the inner man is independent of the body in its existence, it operates in and through the body. When God created mankind He made them in His own image—He breathed in man a pure spirit which was in perfect harmony with the body created from the dust. Man's nature was ethical; he did not even have an inclination to sin. It was, however, possible for him to sin because he had free will. You see, God is a pure and loving God who will not force us to do the things we do not want to do. He directs us to the right path and while He will not force us to take it, He does provide us with the road map and makes Himself available to us should we feel the need to communicate with him. We are free to obey or disobey God, the choice is ours. Adam and Eve used their free will; they chose to obey the devil and disobey God.

When our first parents rebelled against the plan and will of the Creator this harmony was greatly marred—the foundation of that harmony was lost as man died a spiritual death—thus the direct line connecting man to his Creator was severed and the harmony between man's spirit and his flesh was lost. It could be no other way, for man had now freely allowed Satan, the enemy of God, to take abode within him—in essence, man had through his disobedience given the permission of partnership to an evil being that he could not control. Satan was now free to drag in his bag of garbage and flaunt his character. Since that fateful day this has caused a rebellion within man—the rebellion of his lower nature (the flesh) against the higher (the spirit). Man's life on earth became warfare as the flesh, more inclined to seek its own will rather than the will of God, rebelled against the spirit and his higher nature. Galatians 5:17: "**For the flesh lusteth against the Spirit, and the Spirit against the flesh: and these are** contrary the one to the other: so that ye cannot do the things that ye would." God the Creator is an *uncreated* pure Spirit. The angels are *created* pure spirits. A spirit is a being without a body but has an intellect and free will. A pure spirit is one that has no dependence on substance either for its existence or any of its activities.

On the day our first parents yielded to Satan, the tempter, in the Garden of Eden, they died a spiritual death and became separated from God's divine nature. Mankind could no longer communicate with God on the level he was accustomed for the spirit in him had lost connection with the Creator's Spirit. From that day forward the warfare began in man's life as the carnal flesh fought against the spirit for dominance of the body.

The **Carnal Flesh** finds pleasure in the narcissistic activities as documented in Galatians 5:19-21, known as the works of the flesh. These activities are entrenched in the character of Satan, the evil angel whom Adam and Eve chose to obey instead of God.

> "*Now the works of the flesh* are manifest, which are these; *Adultery, fornication, uncleanness, lasciviousness, Idolatry, witchcraft, hatred, variance, emulations, wrath, strife, seditions, heresies, Envyings, murders, drunkenness, revellings,* and such like: of the which I tell you before, as I have also told you in

time past, that they which do such things shall not inherit the kingdom of God." (Galatians 5:19-21) (emphasis added)

The fruit of the Spirit is synonymous with the characteristics of God and is in absolute contrasts to the deeds of the flesh. While the works of the flesh has its foundation in narcissistic conduct and bring pain and suffering to those who embrace the practice as well as those who are caught in the crossfire, the fruit of the Spirit is embedded in altruism and brings peace and happiness to those in its pathway. **"But the fruit of the Spirit is love, joy, peace, longsuffering, gentleness, goodness, faith, Meekness, temperance: against such there is no law."** (Galatians 5:22-23)

On the day Adam and Eve yielded to temptation and rebelled against the plan God had for their lives, they immediately realized that something was different. The Spirit of God had departed from them. Instinctively, they felt the need to replace the spiritual covering that had been stripped away; immediately they leaned to their own understanding and sewed the leaves of fig together for their covering. They realized that they were now unable to stand in the presence of God; a righteous fear had pushed them back so when they heard the voice of God they hid among the trees of the garden—something had come between them and their creator, and they could no longer stay in His presence. It was an experience similar to the one the Israelites had at Sinai when God came down on the mountain. God, being a loving and merciful Father, gave Adam and Eve a blood covering before turning them out of the Garden of Eden. Animals had to be slaughtered to clothe them with the coats of skins—symbolic of the ultimate sacrifice made at Calvary to redeem Adam's fallen race.

> **"And the eyes of them both were opened, and they knew that they were naked; and they sewed fig leaves together, and made themselves aprons. And they heard the voice of the Lord God walking in the garden in the cool of the day: and Adam and his wife hid themselves from the presence of the Lord God amongst the trees of the garden. […] Unto Adam also and to his wife did the Lord God make coats of skins, and clothed them."** (Genesis 3:7, 8, 21)

After the fall, God found new ways to communicate with mankind. We have seen God communicating with man through dreams, through angels, and through his prophets. In Exodus we first saw God communicating with Moses through a burning bush.

In Exodus 19 and 20 we see a divine communication on Mount Sinai between Moses and God Almighty.

Moses was the intermediary between God and the newly emancipated Israelites. God loved these people with an everlasting love but there could be no direct communication because of the void caused by sin which began in the Garden of Eden.

> **"And the Lord said unto Moses, Lo, I come unto thee in a thick cloud, that the people may hear when I speak with thee, and believe thee for ever. And Moses told the words of the people unto the Lord. And the Lord said unto Moses, Go unto the people, and sanctify them to day and to morrow, and let them wash their clothes. And thou shalt set bounds unto the people round about, saying, Take heed to yourselves, that ye go not up into the mount, or touch the border of it: whosoever toucheth the mount shall be surely put to death:"** (Exodus 19:9,10,12)

The people were afraid of the presence of God.

> **"And all the people saw the thunderings, and lightnings, and the noise of the trumpet, and the mountain smoking: and when the people saw it, they removed, and stood afar off. And they said unto Moses, speak thou with us,**

and we will hear: but let not God speak with us, lest we die." (Exodus 20:18-19)

Under Moses we saw God establishing a covenant with Israel (the model nation) and giving them a code of conduct to live by, The Ten Commandments. It was in the covenant of the Law given by Moses that those who would come near to worship the Lord would do so upon an altar made of stone as documented in Exodus 20:25, Leviticus 1-3. We later saw the affirmation of the blood covenant, the Ark of the Covenant and the priestly role of the Levites being established. A communication system between man and God was to remain in place until Jesus, the ultimate sacrifice, was offered up on the cross of Calvary.

The fall of man drastically transformed the entire human existence—life became a struggle as mankind slipped progressively into narcissism and indulged heavily in the works of the flesh. Mankind crossed every boundary, causing the stench of sin to permeate the earth's atmosphere. The Earth became a world where Satan's character flourished everywhere—his signature was on everyone except for one family, the Noah family.

"And it repented the Lord that he had made man on the earth, and it grieved him at his heart. And the Lord said, I will destroy man whom I have created from the face of the earth; both man, and beast, and the

**creeping thing, and the fowls of the air; for
it repenteth me that I have made them."**
(Genesis 6:6-7)

So great was the stench of sin on the earth, God had
to destroy them all by the waters of a flood; leaving only
the Noah family to replenish the earth. We are told in
Genesis 6:9b that Noah was a just man and perfect in his
generations and that he walked with God. It is therefore
not surprising that he was chosen by God to build the ark
prior to the flood, thus, he became the obedient servant
on earth who carried out the will of God. Satan, the
adversary, was not far away; for although all his bodily
agents had been wiped out during the flood, he was not
prepared to give up his long fight for supremacy. Instead,
he waited for an opportune time and when that time was
evident to him he subtly injected sin into Noah's family.
He waited until after the flood, while the earth was being
rebuilt, then he crept into Noah's household.

It is important to note Noah's spiritual strength and
his dedication to his Creator before the flood judgment.
Noah was described as a just man, perfect in his generation
and a man who walked with God and who had found grace
in the eyes of the Lord. Noah was a faithful servant of God
and he had successfully carried out the instructions given
to him by God. It was through his household that the
earth was to be repopulated but in the midst of rebuilding

Satan, the evil angel, showed up at his house and just like he interfered with God's plan in the Garden of Eden he circled Noah's home until he found a weak link through which he could once again interfere with God's plan for humanity.

Here we see Noah and his family, the only humans on earth after the mighty flood. They have worked hard and have started rebuilding their lives. The vineyard Noah planted has flourished—it is a time of plenty and the family has started to feel comfortable. Noah, the head of the household, is fully relaxed and he feels like just taking things easy and enjoying some of that good wine he has produced from his very own vines. He finds the taste of this wine very desirable, and yes, he becomes so self-absorbed that he overindulges until he becomes inebriated and lies in his tent exposed. We all have an idea how impaired the mind of a drunk can be. Many under the influence of alcohol indulge in behavior they would not normally have if alcohol was not a factor. In Proverbs 20:1, Solomon the wise man reminds us that wine is a mocker. Quite often we hear of people who become vulnerable in this state and find themselves open to abusive attacks.

While Noah laid uncovered in the privacy of his tent, Ham, one of his sons, walked in and saw his father's nakedness and then called his two brothers' attention to their father's condition. The two brothers, Shem and

Japheth, unlike Ham choose not to take the immoral pathway. Instead, they honored their father; they walked backward with a garment and covered him. When Noah awoke from his drunken stupor he knew just what his son Ham had done to him and he was very displeased. As a father, he spoke into the lives of his sons. To the two sons who had honored him there was blessing and to the son who had dishonored him, cursing.

It is interesting to note how Satan used self-absorption to open the door to Noah's household—Satan certainly knows how to work the flesh to achieve his aspirations. There is a very important lesson to be learned here. We must realize that Satan is very watchful and persistent and that he is adept at pulling tricks to achieve his purposes. Never think that you are too high up to be touched by Satan. Keep your heart in a state of humbleness, regardless of your position, knowing that you can do nothing without God. Take the emphasis off yourself, walk in humility always, and rely on the Word of God and constant communication through prayer and worship. If God has given you a gift whether it be singing, discerning, healing or being a good public speaker, whatever the case may be, just remember that these are gifts from God; you are a servant, a steward, so don't get entangled in the web of conceit or you will fall very hard.

Once Satan got a toehold in Noah's family, he held on and continued to amplify his character among mankind once again. Egotism and pride was everywhere—man was fully infected. Mankind got to the point where they wanted to make a name for themselves and so they started to build a city and a tower whose top would reach heaven. And just like God had to turn Adam and Eve out of the Garden of Eden for their own good, he also had to confound mankind's language to protect them from their own ignorance, as mankind continued to be influenced by Satan into every imaginable evil."

Subsequently, Satan continued to spread his poison among mankind, craftily encouraging them to defile their bodies and to destroy each other in various ways, thus pushing them further and further away from their Creator and Father, God Almighty.

One thing is clear, wherever Satan is there is strife, and there is grief and pain for the victims—that's a constant. The old serpent that he is, he takes a convoluted course slithering, gliding, turning, twisting, curling up, and stirring up trouble—as he plants the poisonous seed then conceals himself and watches with delight as his victim(s) takes the bait and suffers the consequence(s). He then waits for the right time to strike again. Satan is the chief enemy of God and mankind. He has worked tirelessly to create an abyss between man and God but he is now a defeated foe since Jesus bridged that gap by taking on the sins of mankind and dying on the cross at Calvary. In the Garden of Gethsemane Jesus took on our sins, taking back from Satan what he stole from mankind in the Garden of Eden. The character of Satan the deceiver has been unmasked and it is now up to you and me to decide whether we will continue to be tricked by the adversary or choose to keep our eyes on Christ, the Redeemer, who conquered this evil angel called Satan to give us the opportunity for a new life. The new life we should have had when God wiped out the agents of Satan and repopulated the earth with Noah's family who also, like Adam and Eve, proved a failure when they allowed Satan entry into their household.

The bible tells us in Luke 22:43-44 that Jesus prayed earnestly in the Garden of Gethsemane because He was in agony; He prayed until His sweat was like great drops of blood. So great was the agony that an angel was sent from heaven to strengthen Him. It was a very severe mental anguish as He struggled victoriously—taking on the severely flawed character of Adam's fallen race in His own body. The burden of the sin of the world was so great that He fell along the Via Dela Rosa. On the cross He felt rejection as he carried the sins of mankind and He called out to His Father: "My God, My God, Why hast thou forsaken me?" In spite of the excruciating physical and emotional pain Jesus suffered, He completed man's redemption at Calvary—His last words were: **"It is finished."**

The order and harmony lost in the Garden of Eden could not be restored through the blood of animals. Animal blood could only serve as a temporary covering but today mankind has a permanent covering through Jesus the Christ who died on the cross at Calvary for the remission of our transgressions. If we are willing to accept the redemptive work done at Calvary, we can restore that order and harmony in our individual lives for Christ gave us newness of life when he took our old nature to the cross. We have been made new in Christ, all we have to do is accept His gift and by so doing take on His character and a new life. **"For as in Adam all die, even so in Christ shall all be made alive."** (1 Cor. 15:22) Simply stated, the good news is that Christ through his death on the cross of Calvary has made it possible for the harmony between the flesh and spirit to be fully restored.

"I am crucified with Christ: nevertheless I live; yet not I, but Christ liveth in me: and the life which I now live in the flesh I live by the faith of the Son of God, who loved me, and gave himself for me." (Galatians 2:20) The body (flesh) is ordained for dissolution but the soul (spirit being) is immortal, so let us forsake the work of the flesh and walk in obedience taking on the fruit of the spirit as we embrace our new life in Christ Jesus.

"Let this mind be in you, which was also in Christ Jesus:"
(Philippians 2:5)

The Tongue at a Glance

Physically, the tongue is a small organ but it is resilient as it is productive. It talks, mixes food, swallows, tastes and fights germs. Even when we are sleeping our tongue is busy pushing saliva into the throat to be swallowed—it never gets a rest. Over a lifetime the average person will suffer impairment of the eyes, ears, teeth, lungs, kidney, heart, etc. which often lead to corrective measures being implemented respectively. The tongue, however, regardless of its physical condition generally stays with us until we depart this life. I have never heard of any tongue being **successfully** transplanted to carry out all the functions God created it to perform.

In 2003, surgeons at Vienna's General Hospital in Austria performed the first ever tongue transplant surgery on a human being. The operation lasted 14 hours but at the end of the surgery the surgeon who headed the team said that it was unlikely the sense of taste would be restored; he was, however, hopeful that with the new tongue, harvested from an accident victim, the patient would be able to talk and eat as normal—hope was all he could give. Also, there was a high risk of infection because the mouth is a non-sterile environment. According to doctors, conventionally, in cases where patients lose their tongues, surgeons would remove a minute piece of their small intestines and graft that onto the tongue stump. Such patients, however, were never able to speak clearly or swallow again, and must be fed through tubes.

Just think of the many things we would not be able to do if we had no tongue. We would not be able to enjoy our favorite foods for the tongue is made up of many groups of muscles which run in different directions to carry out the jobs designated for the tongue. The front of the tongue is very lithe and can move around the mouth with ease and comfort as it works with the teeth to create a multitude of words. This part of the tongue also helps us eat by moving the food around our mouth while we chew. The tongue pushes the food to the back teeth so the teeth can grind it up.

Chinese medicine practitioners believe the appearance of the tongue can reveal a lot about one's health. It is said that the normal tongue color is light red and that this color indicates a person's vital energy is strong. According to practitioners in Chinese alternative medicine, it also reflects the health of the internal organs and blood circulation—changes in the tongue color usually reflect chronic illness.

In his evaluation of the tongue, James the Apostle rightly sums up this small organ which is so imperative to our speech. James draws a parallel between the bits placed in the horse's mouth, the helm of a ship, and the human tongue. He noted that the whole body of the horse is controlled by the bits placed in its mouth and likewise a ship, though huge and driven by fierce wind, is controlled by a very small helm. Yet the tongue, a diminutive member, cannot be tamed by man. It is an unruly evil full of deadly poison. It is capable of being boastful as well as being destructive to the highest level—like a small fire it can ignite its target and cause vast devastation.

> **"Behold, we put bits in the horses' mouths, that they may obey us; and we turn about their whole body. Behold also the ships, which though they be so great, and are driven of fierce winds, yet are they turned about with a very small helm, Withersover the governor listeth. Even so the tongue is a little member, and boasteth great things. Behold, how great a matter a little fire kindleth! But the tongue can no man tame; it is an unruly evil, full of deadly poison."**
> (James 3:3-5, 8)

So often we hear of massive forest fires burning out of control for days, destroying wildlife, public, and private properties as well as taking the lives of those who fight to bring them under control. By the time these fires are brought under control they have stretched the resources of communities and forever changed the lives of many in different ways. These fires are generally ignited by a spark from a source and quickly gain momentum leaving in its path overwhelming devastation which can take a lifetime to rebuild. This is exactly the type of damage equated with the tongue—a very scary realization especially when we know the tongue was not intended to be a deadly weapon.

Although the tongue was never meant to be used unconstructively, since the fall of mankind it has been used as a destructive weapon in every generation—ruthlessly wounding, maiming, and plundering the unsuspecting victim. The tongue like every other member of our body was made by God for a specific purpose and was intended to be used in the approved manner. Apart from the uses as mentioned earlier, the tongue should be used in worshipping God, the Creator. Colossians 1:16-17 states: **"For by Him were all things created, that are in heaven, and that are in the earth, visible and invisible, whether they be thrones, or dominions, or principalities, or powers: all**

**things were created by Him, and for Him: And he is
before all things, and by him all things consist."**

James describes the tongue as an unruly evil, full of
deadly poison. He further declares that no man can tame
the tongue. James has painted an accurate picture of an
ungodly tongue—a tongue being manipulated as a weapon
of Satan, a flesh-driven tongue—being in subjection to the
flesh rather than the spirit. The tongue can only be tamed
by God who through his mercy and goodness to a fallen
people sent his Son, Jesus Christ, to redeem us through his
saving grace at the cross of Calvary.

The ungodly tongue is the extension of a mutinous
heart in rebellion against God and His handiwork and
seeks to take control at any cost. The ungodly tongue is the
mirror of a heart in rebellion; it reflects the intent of the
heart. How many times have we heard people say 'oops, I
didn't mean that. It came out the wrong way.' I say to you,
that was exactly what you meant. You did not intend to
give anybody a glimpse of what was hiding in your heart
but your mirror, the tongue, reflected it—too late now.

The Word of God says:

> **"The heart is deceitful above all things,
> and desperately wicked: who can know it?"**
> (Jeremiah 17:9)

"A good man out of the good treasure of his heart bringeth forth that which is good; and an evil man out of the evil treasure of his heart bringeth forth that which is evil: for of the abundance of the heart his mouth speaketh." (Luke 6:45)

"Let the high praises of God be in their mouth,
and a twoedged sword in their hand;"
(Psalm 149:6)

The Adversary

*"From whence come wars and fightings among you?
Come they not hence, even of your lusts that war in your
members? Ye lust, and have not: ye kill, and desire to
have, and cannot obtain: ye fight and war, yet ye have not,
because ye ask not. Ye adulterers and adulteresses, know
ye not that the friendship of the world is enmity with
God? whosoever therefore will be a friend of the world is
an enemy of God."* **Do ye think that the scripture saith in
vain, The spirit that dwelleth in us lusteth to envy?"**
(James 4:1-2, 4-5)

We live in a world dominated by suffering. Popular
mediums such as television, radio and Internet stream
images and sounds directly to us. Without even leaving
our homes we come face to face with suffering—war torn
and poverty stricken countries, local and international
crimes, broken families, economic distress, and diseases
of all sorts. All of this suffering that has been showered
on mankind have a common source—sin. "Where did this

sin originate?" This is a question many ask from time to time. The answer to this question is: Sin originated with an evil angel now known by several names but the most popular among these names are: Satan, the devil, and the adversary.

Satan did not begin his life as an evil angel. He was a very beautiful and talented angel called Lucifer who held a very important position in heaven. But after a while he became self-absorbed and decided that he could be a better ruler than God his Creator—he had a desire for honor and supremacy and he went to war against his Creator in an effort to gain that status. Lucifer started a rebellion in heaven and was able to convince one-third of the angels in heaven to join him—what persuasive power. Satan lost the rebellion he started and as a result he and the angels who joined him in the rebellion were thrown out of heaven. The prophets of God Isaiah and Ezekiel gave an account of Lucifer, his job and privilege in heaven and his fall from the heavenly realm:

> **"How art thou fallen from heaven, O Lucifer, son of the morning! how art thou cut down to the ground, which didst weaken the nations! For thou hast said in thine heart, I will ascend into heaven, I will exalt my throne above the stars of God: I will sit also upon the mount of the congregation, in the**

sides of the north: I will ascend above the heights of the clouds; I will be like the most High." (Isaiah 14:12-14)

"Thus saith the Lord God; Thou sealest up the sum, full of wisdom and perfect in beauty. Thou has been in Eden the garden of God; every precious stone was thy covering, the sardius, topaz, and the diamond, the beryl, the onyx, and the jasper, the sapphire, the emerald, and the carbuncle, and gold: the workmanship of thy tabrets and of thy pipes was prepared in thee in the day that thou was created. Thou art the anointed cherub that covereth; and I have set thee so: thou wast upon the holy mountain of God; thou has walked up and down in the midst of the stones of fire. Thou wast perfect in thy ways from the day that thou was created, till iniquity was found in thee. By the multitude of thy merchandise they have filled the midst of thee with violence, and thou hast sinned: therefore I will cast thee as profane out of the mountain of God: and I will destroy thee, O covering cherub, from the midst of the stones of fire. Thine heart was lifted up because of thy beauty, thou hast corrupted

thy wisdom by reason of thy brightness: I will cast thee to the ground, I will lay thee before kings, that they may behold thee. Thou has defiled thy sanctuaries by the multitude of thine iniquities, by the iniquity of thy traffick; therefore will I bring forth a fire from the midst of thee, it shall devour thee, and I will bring thee to ashes upon the earth in the sight of all them that behold thee." (Ezekiel 28:12b-18)

When Satan the rebel, the deceiver, the liar lost the war he initiated in heaven, he also lost his home and rank there but he did not humble himself; he could have gone to any other corner on the earth and settled but that was not his intention. His intention was to continue his attack against God and His plan for mankind so he walked into the beautiful home of a couple, a home where there was abundance, harmony, and the peace that passes all understanding—this was the happy home of Adam and Eve, his wife. When he entered he only came to steal and destroy to serve his own self-centered purpose. He knew if he could only get them to disobey God he would get a foot in the door. He would have won the right to claim them as his own, for in fact, they would be in contravention of God's command just like Satan himself who had been thrown out of heaven for this same reason. There, Satan disguised himself in the body of the serpent and cunningly sowed the seed of lust in Eve's heart causing her to yearn for the fruit which she had been told by God never to eat. Satan knew that if he could only get them to eat the fruit they would lose their home and the comfort it provided and in the long run he would benefit. Like a defence lawyer he posed his question to Eve and watched with delight as she tripped and fell. In that moment, the old serpent knew he had shrewdly stolen from Adam and Eve—dominion over the earth, the authority God had given them, was now in the hand of Satan.

> **"And he said unto the woman, Yea, hath God said, Ye shall not eat of every tree of the garden?**
>
> **And the woman said unto the serpent, We may eat of the fruit of the trees of the garden: But of the fruit of the tree which is in the midst of the garden, God hath said, Ye shall not eat of it, neither shall ye touch it, lest ye die.**
>
> **And the serpent said unto the woman, Ye shall not surely die: For God doth know that in the day ye eat thereof, then your eyes shall**

be opened, and ye shall be as gods, knowing good and evil." (Genesis 3:1b-5)

The tactic used by Satan in getting Eve's attention is very significant and I must point out that he still uses this tactic today. He started his conversation with Eve by questioning God's instruction to Adam and Eve—thus sowing a seed of doubt in her heart. The next thing he did was to reinforce that doubt and continue to build on that doubt until she developed a desire and yielded to the temptation. **"And when the woman saw that the tree was good for food, and that it was pleasant to the eyes, and a tree to be desired to make one wise, she took of the fruit thereof, and did eat, and gave also unto her husband with her; and he did eat."** (Genesis 3:6)

Since that day Satan has crossed many boundaries. He took dominion over earth and inaugurated his fight against mankind. No longer did Satan limit himself to using the serpent's body to perpetrate his diabolical plots but he commenced using mankind against mankind. Abel was the first of Satan's casualty when he was killed by Cain, his own brother, in the open fields. When God asked Cain for his brother he answered with a tongue that was rude and full of lies and deception: "Am I my brother's keeper?" Here we see Cain being possessed by the character of Satan—jealousy, rebellion, malice, pride, murder, arrogance, and lies. **"And Cain talked with Abel** his brother: and it came to pass, when they were in the field, that Cain rose up against Abel his brother, and slew him. And the Lord said unto Cain, Where is Abel thy brother? And he said I know not: Am I my brother's keeper?" (Genesis 4:8-9)

I believe that this was a profound period of grief for Adam and Eve for on that day they lost both sons. Cain's life became more difficult, not only did he have to live under *the family curse* but he also had to live under his own curse—he had to face the consequence of his action.

> "And he said, What hast thou done? the voice of thy brother's blood crieth unto me from the ground. And now art thou cursed from the earth, which hath opened her mouth to receive thy brother's blood from thy hand; When thou tillest the ground, it shall not henceforth yield unto thee her strength; a fugitive and a vagabond shalt thou be in the earth. And Cain said unto the Lord, My punishment is greater than I can bear." (Genesis 4:10-13)

Let us stop for a minute and think of the many people who are being killed each day through wars, gang violence on the streets, and violence in the home. Many of these victims might not have known Christ as their personal savior, and so, might have died in their fallen state before accepting the saving grace provided by Jesus at the cross of Calvary. When this happens another soul is added to the adversary's camp to await judgment.

Violence hurts victims and perpetrators as well as their families and dependants. The emotional and financial loss can be very devastating causing families to lose their homes and general standard of living. So often when these situations play out we blame the perpetrator, the one who is tangible, for we cannot see the one who has possessed the perpetrator. The Apostle Paul had many revelations from God and this is what he said to the Ephesians: **"For we wrestle not against flesh and blood, but against principalities, against powers, against the rulers of the darkness of this world, against spiritual wickedness in high places."** (Ephesians 6:12)

The world is continually under the attack of Satan, the adversary, as he continues his struggle for supremacy against his Creator and the souls of mankind. It is a warfare, a conflict that will persist to the end and every one of us is engaged in it and so the church needs to keep praying for the salvation of those who are still being used by the adversary to commit various levels of discord against mankind. We also need to keep the devil out of our homes and communities by using the weapons Christ has given us as believers. **"The effectual fervent prayer of a righteous man availeth much."** (James 5:16b)

During Christ's journey on earth, He was attacked by the adversary numerous times but Christ recognized the demonic attack and used the Word of God against Satan. Satan was never able to penetrate the mind of Christ—from the temptations in the wilderness as documented in Matthew 4:1-11 to the final attempt to persuade Christ to come down from the cross. Satan was resolute in his attack on Christ's earthly ministry but not even by a thought did Christ yield to that rebel angel. Peter and Judas, both disciples of Jesus Christ, were used by Satan against Him.

Let's take a look at how Satan used the unwitting Peter against Jesus as He began to reveal the scope of His mission to the disciples: **"From that time forth began Jesus to show His disciples, how that He must go unto Jerusalem, and suffer many things of the elders and chief priests and scribes, and be killed, and raised again the third day."** (Matthew 16:21)

Peter took Jesus aside and said to Him, **"Be it far from thee, Lord: this shall not be unto thee."** (Matthew 16:22b) Peter loved Jesus and his objective was to protect Jesus but he was innocently being used by Satan to hinder the redemptive purpose of God. Since that day in the Garden of Eden when man sinned and was separated from God, man took on the characteristics of Satan who now knows how to shrewdly use these traits in mankind to accomplish his purpose. Satan tempts mankind through: pride, carnality, and selfishness which he knows is naturally embedded in man's character. Here we see Peter leaning to his own understanding, extending to Jesus self-assurance, showing dependence on his own egocentricity to bring into play man-made plans. This was the same kind of behavior Sarah encouraged when she doubted God's promise and formulated a carnal plan in which Abraham allowed himself to be led into having a child by Hagar, Sarah's maid—it was to be a costly error, which still to this day has plagued the fruit of Sarah's womb. Eve was the one to throw this door wide open for Satan to walk through, when she took on carnality through her desire for the forbidden fruit. Jesus, recognizing that the devil was operating through Peter, immediately rebuked him saying, **"Get thee behind me, Satan: thou art an offence unto me: for thou savourest not the things that be of God, but those that be of men."** (Matthew 16:23) Jesus later said to Peter, **"Simon, Simon, behold, Satan hath desired to have you, that he may sift you as wheat: But I have prayed for thee, that thy faith fail not: and when thou art converted, strengthen thy brethren."** (Luke 22:31-32)

Just take a look at the world around you. There are so many businesses that have been started by people who at one time or another had worked with a company and through that employment became privy to information which they later used to successfully start a similar business of their own—Satan since his fall from heaven has utilized this same ploy. Satan is a very gifted spirit being; as Lucifer, he was once a resident of heaven so he knows just how to read certain signs. He has continued to use his gift and the information to which he was privy, as a good angel called Lucifer, to wreak havoc in the world at large. In the Garden of Eden after the fall of man, God said to him: **"And I will put enmity between thee and the woman, and between they seed and her seed; it shall bruise thy head, and thou shalt bruise his heel."** (Genesis 3:15)

Satan has not forgotten any of this and that is the reason he tried to kill Moses, the baby. Satan used Pharaoh to make and enforce a law that all boys born to the Hebrew women should be put to death. Satan knew that a baby of prominence would be born during this time but he did not know the exact baby so he made the ruling to kill every baby so there would be no chance for this special baby to escape. Satan was not able to destroy this baby who was to be used by God in many ways to bring mankind closer to Him. It was through this baby that the Ten Commandments and the Pentateuch, the first five books of the bible, were given. As well, Jesus the redeemer of Adam's fallen race came out of the people Moses led from bondage in Egypt.

Again, when Jesus was born Satan knew that a special baby had come into the world and he used King Herod, as his agent, to give command to kill all the boy babies two years old and under in and around Bethlehem, hoping he would destroy the **'Promised Baby'.** Satan knew the importance of this baby but again he was not able to hurt this baby.

Satan never gave up and finally he used the disciple Judas Iscariot, who had a weakness for financial gains, to betray Christ in exchange for money. As Christ hung dead on the Roman cross, Satan was happy; he thought he had successfully obstructed the redemption of Adam's fallen race for ever. He felt he had once again derailed God's plan for humanity; but the victory Satan thought he had was short-lived— the empty tomb three days later proved to be Satan's worst defeat. It meant that the devil was conquered; all that he had taken from Adam and Eve had been restored to their ancestors—the doors were flung open to the "whosoever will". **"For God so loved the world, that he gave his only begotten Son, that whosoever believeth in him should not perish, but have everlasting life."** (John 3:16)

One does not have to be demon possessed to be used by Satan and that is the reason we need to be on guard less we inadvertently allow the devil to use us. It's no wonder

Paul admonished us to pray without ceasing—prayer paralyzes Satan.

Today, so many happy and stable homes are destroyed because some agent of the devil entices a member of that family to try a substance or an act. The typical line is: 'Try it once and if you don't like it...'' So often many addictions or bad habits are picked up in this way whether it is related to drugs, alcohol, gambling, extra-marital affair, or first-time fornication. Many unplanned pregnancies and venereal diseases, even the dreaded AIDS and HIV are, quite often, a result of such temptations. When these strongholds enter ones life it causes great suffering for everyone involved.

It is important to remember that Satan, the adversary of man's salvation, is the master of deceit and that he never presents both sides of a story. He is adept at covering and marketing sin in the most appealing packages you will ever find. He directs the operation making sure you see only what he wants you to see—the fun and the excitement, the look-good and the feel-good elements are accentuated. Consequences and long-term effects are kept in the dark and only *you* will suffer after you have taken the alluring bate. History has repeated itself so many times in generation after generation but the lessons are never learned for Satan is so good at his game; it is hard to see the concealed poison he carries, it is only after the fact when the persuasive adversary has left that we realize the error in judgment. Since the fall of man, Satan has seized and overshadowed the world in a deceitful clasp of lies, suffering and death. Satan sells a product that is poisonous and heavily saturated with sin—a rejection of God, the Creator of the universe. He never stops peddling this merchandise; he presents his product in various attractive packages making it enticing and inviting to the unsuspecting victim—just as he did in the Garden of Eden. Satan's tricks are not new; they are simply concealed in an assortment of attractive packages, but just like Christ we will be able to recognize the adversary if we walk in the spirit. **"For the eyes of the Lord are over the righteous, and His ears are open unto their prayers: But the face of the Lord is against them that do evil."** (1 Peter 3:12)

"Be sober, be vigilant; because your adversary the devil,
as a roaring lion, walketh about,
seeking whom he may devour:"

(1 Peter 5:8)

The Heart

"Keep thy heart with all diligence;
for out of it are the issues of life". (Proverbs 4:23)

The wise man Solomon understood that the heart is the core of morality and the wellspring of deeds, and although he did not guard his own heart he was sensible enough to put his knowledge in writing to serve as a warning to those who would come after him.

The heart of man is indeed his worst element before it is rehabilitated and the best after transformation has taken place. In its rebellious state the heart is exceedingly wicked and deceitful above all things; no man can know the deep dark recesses of the heart but the eyes of God are always on the heart of man. When Samuel was sent to Bethlehem by the Lord for the purpose of anointing one of Jesse's sons to be king of Israel, his first impression when he laid eyes on Eliab was that this was the son to be anointed but the Lord spoke to him saying, "**Look not on his countenance, or on the height of his stature; because I have refused him:**

for the Lord seeth not as man seeth; for man looketh on the outward appearance, but the Lord looketh on the heart." (1 Samuel 16:7)

The heart is the area where Satan creeps in and plants his sin-laden seeds, then leaves it to develop into various ungodly products. An evil heart is not developed overnight, it evolves over time as the poisonous seeds take root and mature. It can be very overwhelming to see just how frigid the human heart is capable of becoming when it surrenders itself to evil schemes. God hates a heart that deviseth wicked imaginations and feet that are swift in running to mischief. An evil heart brings pain and suffering to others and, like an unpredictable cat brought home from the wild as a pet, it will eventually turn on its owner in a destructive rampage.

Our thought life should be acceptable to God for the area of our thoughts is the battlefield—it is here that the warfare begins before crossing into other areas of our lives. If we purpose within our hearts to win the battle here, then we will rejoice in the victory God gives us over the enemy daily. Thoughts are Satan's strongholds, the wicked imaginations found there are from him and we must pull them down with the Word of God—**"For the weapons of our warfare are not carnal, but mighty through God to the pulling down of strong holds;"** (2 Corinthians 10:4)

"For they that are after the flesh do mind the things of the flesh; but they that are after the Spirit the things of the Spirit." (Romans 8:5)

"Ye shall know them by their fruits. Do men gather grapes of thorns, or figs of thistles? Even so every good tree bringeth forth good fruit; but a corrupt tree bringeth forth evil fruit. A good tree cannot bring forth evil fruit, neither can a corrupt tree bring forth good fruit." (Matthew 7:16-18)

Although slightly larger than a clenched fist, the heart is a very powerful muscle located in the center of the chest. It works as a pump, sending blood laden with oxygen and nutrients throughout the body. The oxygen-rich blood travels throughout the arteries and vessels, nourishing the body so it can function properly. The heart will beat an average of 100,000 times per day and would have pumped more than 4,300 gallons of blood throughout the entire body during that time.

The heart has four chambers—two at the top (the atria) and two at the bottom (the ventricles). The heart's only function is to pump blood. The right side of the heart pumps blood to the lungs, where oxygen is added to the blood and carbon dioxide is removed from it. The left side pumps blood to the rest of the body, where oxygen and nutrients are delivered to tissues and waste products (such as carbon dioxide) are transferred to the blood for removal by other organs (such as the lungs and kidneys).

As I look at the intricate function of this small organ that is so essential to the human existence, I am reminded of God's command to the Israelites being led by Moses through the wilderness—**"Moreover ye shall eat no manner of blood, whether it be of fowl or of beast, in any of your dwellings. Whatsoever soul it be that eateth any manner of blood, even that soul shall be cut off from his people."** (Leviticus 7:26-27)

"Only be sure that thou eat not the blood: for the blood is the life; and thou mayest not eat the life with the flesh" (Deuteronomy 12:23)

I continue to marvel at the mysteries of God. The blood, the life, is regulated by the heart, the nucleus of the body. God keeps his eyes on this oracle where both the physical and spiritual well being of the complete person is focused. If tainted blood is pumped through this organ to the body, the body cells will eventually die. If evil is planted in the heart and allowed to flourish, it will certainly result in spiritual death to the owner and many lives will no doubt be destroyed as the poison is spewed out of the tongue and other members of the body. In the end there will be severe consequences—the Word of God declares:

> **"For the wicked boasteth of his heart's desire, and blesseth the covetous, whom**

the Lord abhorreth. The wicked, through the pride of his countenance, will not seek after God: God is not in all his thoughts. His ways are always grievous; thy judgments are far above out of his sight: as for all his enemies, he puffeth at them. He hath said in his heart, I shall never be moved: for I shall never be in adversity. His mouth is full of cursing and deceit and fraud: under his tongue is mischief and vanity. He sitteth in the lurking places of the villages: in the secret places doth he murder the innocent: his eyes are privily set against the poor. He lieth in wait secretly as a lion in his den: he lieth in wait to catch the poor: he doth catch the poor, when he draweth him into his net. He croucheth, and humbleth himself, that the poor may fall by his strong ones. He hath said in his heart, God hath forgotten: he hideth his face; he will never see it." (Psalm 10:3-11)

In my research, I found that Chinese medicine links the tongue with the heart (Kaptchuk 2000, 89). Chinese medicine asserts that the heart governs the blood vessels, houses the mind and spirit, and opens into the tongue. The tongue is considered to be the sprout of the heart—

relating specifically to the tip of the tongue, but it also influences the color, form, and appearance of the tongue. The sense of taste is controlled by the heart; therefore, disease of the heart can easily be recognized on the tongue. Speech is also directly affected by the heart (i.e., stutters, aphasia). If the heart is weak and blood is deficient the tongue will be pale and thin. If the heart is in excess there may be excessive or inappropriate laughter, states of over-joy, and non-stop talking.

Researchers at Penn State College of Medicine have also linked the tongue to the heart (Zahner, Li, and Chen *2003)*. Researchers have found evidence suggesting that the same type of nerve receptors that register the burning sensation from hot peppers in the mouth may cause the sensation of chest pain from a heart attack. This research was funded by the National Heart, Lung, and Blood Institute of the National Institutes of Health. For those of us who know that the Word of God, among other things, is also a compass for mankind we are not surprise when science proves what we already know—there are numerous references in the Bible linking the tongue with the heart. This is overwhelming proof that God's Word is accurate and we are a created people and not a people who evolved over time.

In responding to the religious zealots of His day, Scribes and Pharisees, Jesus said:

O generation of vipers, how can ye being evil, speak good things? for out of the abundance of the heart the mouth speaketh. (Matthew 12:34)

But those things which proceed out of the mouth come forth from the heart; and they defile the man. For out of the heart proceed evil thoughts, murders, adulteries, fornications, thefts, false witness, blasphemies. (Matthew 15:18-19)

For from within, out of the heart of men, proceed evil thoughts, adulteries, fornications, murders. (Mark 7:21)

A good man out of the good treasure of his heart bringeth forth that which is good; and an evil man out of the evil treasure of his heart bringeth forth that which is evil: for of the abundance of the heart his mouth speaketh. (Luke 6:45)

It is no wonder that David, after his adulterous relationship with Bath-sheba, the wife of Uriah (2 Samuel 11 and 12), cried out to God as recorded in Psalm 51:10, *"Create in me a clean heart, O God; and renew a right spirit within me."*

David learned a lot from this costly mistake, hence, he made a conscious effort to walk in uprightness before God:

> **"I said, I will take heed to my ways, that I sin not with my tongue: I will keep my mouth with a bridle, while the wicked is before me."** (Psalm 39:1)

> **"Set a watch, O Lord, before my mouth; keep the door of my lips. Incline not my heart to any evil thing, to practise wicked works with men that work iniquity: and let me not eat of their dainties."** (Psalm 141:3-4)

In Deuteronomy 10:16 we read: **"Circumcise therefore the foreskin of your heart, and be no more stiffnecked."** Circumcision is cutting away of the flesh. It is imperative for mankind to submit to the spirit and not the flesh. Spiritually, circumcision is the renewal of the mind, which allows us to stay clear of the natural, sinful, Adamic nature we are born with. It indicates that the old nature, with its immoral desires, and thought patterns have been obliterated and we now listen to and obey the Holy Spirit.

The human heart in its uncircumcised state can be a toxic cesspool; it represents uncleanness and thus becomes a playground for Satan, a venomous pit where every evil plot is hatched. The heart is not visible but the words volleyed from the tongue reflect the state of the heart.

It is time to stop Satan in his track; renew your mind with the sword of the Spirit, the Word of God, and allow the Holy Spirit to remove the unwanted nature of your flesh, that you may enter into a profound relationship with God. Paul in his letter to the church in Rome and Corinth said:

> **I Beseech you therefore, brethren, by the mercies of God, that ye present your bodies a living sacrifice, holy, acceptable unto God, which is your reasonable service. And be not conformed to this world: but be ye transformed by the renewing of your mind, that ye may prove what is that good, and acceptable, and perfect will of God. (Romans 12:1-2)**

> **For though we walk in the flesh, we do not war after the flesh: For the weapons of our warfare are not carnal, but mighty through God to the pulling down of strong holds: Casting down imaginations, and every high thing that exalteth itself against the knowledge of God, and bringing into captivity every thought to the obedience of**

Christ; And having in a readiness to revenge all disobedience, when your obedience is fulfilled. (2 Corinthians 10:3-6)

"Know ye not that ye are the temple of God, and that the Spirit of God dwelleth in you?" If any man defile the temple of God, him shall God destroy; for the temple of God is holy, which temple ye are." (1 Corinthians 3:16-17)

The Tongue as a Servant

"The Lord God hath given me the tongue of the learned,
that I should know how to speak a word in season to
him that is weary: he wakeneth mine ear to hear as the
learned." (Isaiah 50:4)

There are those who see the tongue as a necessary evil, this is a grave misconception. Every member of our body was created by God, the creator of the universe, for a purpose—only good gifts come from God. David in communing with God the Almighty said, **"I will praise thee; for I am fearfully and wonderfully made: marvellous are thy works; and that my soul knoweth right well."** (Psalm 139:14)

In a fallen world where Satan, the self-proclaimed prince of this world, wrestles for sovereignty it is imperative that the tongue operates as a servant rather than a master. The fundamental attribute and focus of a servant is **humility.** A servant realizes that the Master and His will are primary—without the master I can do nothing.

<u>The servant **seeks the Master**</u> and waits for His revelation.

> "Howbeit when he, the Spirit of truth, is come, he will guide you into all truth: for he shall not speak of himself; but whatsoever he shall hear, that shall he speak: and he will shew you things to come." (John 16:13)

> "…lean not unto thine own understanding." (Proverbs 3:5b)

> "If ye continue in my word, then are ye my disciples indeed; And ye shall know the truth, and the truth shall make you free." (John 8:31b-32)

> "And I say unto you, Ask, and it shall be given you; seek, and ye shall find; knock, and it shall be opened unto you. For every one that asketh receiveth; and he that seeketh findeth; and to him that knocketh it shall be opened." (Luke 11: 9-10)

> "But seek ye first the kingdom of God, and His righteousness; and all these things shall be added unto you." (Matthew 6:33)

The servant **loves the Master** and shows this love through obedience—it is in obedience that deeper knowledge is gained.

> "**If ye love me, keep my commandments. And I will pray the Father, and he shall give you another Comforter, that he may abide with you forever;**" (John 14:15-16)

> "**My sheep hear my voice, and I know them, and they follow me:**" (John 10:27)

> "**By this shall all men know that ye are my disciples, if ye have love one to another.**" (John 13:35)

> "**If any man serve me, let him follow me; and where I am, there shall also my servant be: if any man serve me, him will my Father honour.**" (John 12:26)

> "**Then shall we know, if we follow on to know the Lord: his going forth is prepared as the morning; and he shall come unto us as the rain, as the latter and former rain unto the earth.**" (Hosea 6:3)

> "**If ye keep my commandments, ye shall abide in my love; even as I have kept my**

Father's commandments, and abide in his love." (John 15:10)

The servant **serves the Master** in service to others.

"And Jesus said unto them, Come ye after me, and I will make you to become fishers of men. And straightway they forsook their nets, and followed him." (Mark 1:17-18)

"And he that reapeth receiveth wages, and gathereth fruit unto life eternal: that both he that soweth and he that reapeth may rejoice together." (John 4:36)

"Herein is my Father glorified, that ye bear much fruit; so shall ye be my disciples." (John 15:8)

"But Jesus called them to him, and saith unto them, Ye know that they which are accounted to rule over the Gentiles exercise lordship over them; and their great ones exercise authority upon them. But so shall it not be among you: but whosoever will be great among you, shall be your minister: And whosoever of you will be the chiefest, shall be servant of all. For even the Son of man came not to be ministered unto, but to minister, and to give his life a ransom for many." (Mark 10:42-45)

"Then saith He unto His disciples, The harvest truly is plenteous, but the labourers are few; Pray ye therefore the Lord of the harvest, that He will send forth labourers into His harvest." (Matthew 9:37-38)

"If I then, your Lord and Master, have washed your feet; ye also ought to wash one another's feet." (John 13:14)

The servant **exalts the Master** as he glorifies Him.

"For ye are bought with a price: therefore glorify God in your body, and in your spirit, which are God's." (1 Corinthians 6:20)

"Serve the Lord with gladness: come before his presence with singing." (Psalm 100:2)

"And when they were come to him, he said unto them, Ye know, from the first day that I came into Asia, after what manner I have been with you at all seasons, Serving the Lord with all humility of mind, and with many tears, and temptations, which befell me by the lying in wait of the Jews:" (Acts 20:18-19)

"Herein is my Father glorified, that ye bear much fruit; so shall ye be my disciples." (John 15:8)

The servant is **accountable to the Master.**

"And that servant, which knew his Lord's will, and prepared not himself, neither did according to his will, shall be beaten with many stripes." (Luke 12:47)

"Knowing that of the Lord ye shall receive the reward of the inheritance: for ye serve the Lord Christ." (Colossians 3:24)

"And now, Israel, what doth the Lord thy God require of thee, but to fear the Lord thy God, to walk in all his ways, and to love him, and to serve the Lord thy God with all thy heart and with all thy soul." (Deuteronomy 10:12)

"I delight to do thy will, O my God: yea, thy law is within my heart." (Psalm 40:8)

"Then spake Jesus again unto them, saying, I am the light of the world: he that followeth me shall not walk in darkness, but shall have the light of life." (John 8:12)

Mankind was created to worship God, the Creator. The tongue was meant to be a servant submitting to the higher nature of the spirit. Let your tongue be transformed into an instrument of praise and honour to God the Almighty and a tool of encouragement and kindness to your fellow man. You must never forget the role of the servant in relation to the Master—the first and foremost purpose of the tongue is to praise and worship God through prayers, songs, and the proclamation of His word—we are clearly instructed in His words to do so.

> **"Make a joyful noise unto the Lord, all ye lands.**
>
> **Serve the Lord with gladness: come before his presence with singing.**
>
> **Know ye that the Lord he is God: it is he that hath made us, and not we ourselves; we are his people, and the sheep of his pasture.**
>
> **Enter into his gates with thanksgiving, and into his courts with praise: be thankful unto him, and bless his name.**
>
> **For the Lord is good; his mercy is everlasting; and his truth endureth to all generations."**
> (Psalm 100)

"Even every one that is called by my name: for I have created him for my glory, I have formed him; yea, I have made him." (Isaiah 43:7)

"This people have I formed for myself; they shall shew forth my praise." (Isaiah 43:21)

"All nations whom thou hast made shall come and worship before thee, O Lord; and shall glorify thy name." (Psalms 86:9)

"Let every thing that hath breath praise the Lord. Praise ye the Lord." (Psalms 150:6)

"For mine own sake, even for mine own sake, will I do it: for how should my name be polluted? and I will not give my glory unto another." (Isaiah 48:11)

"In every thing give thanks: for this is the will of God in Christ Jesus concerning you." (1 Thessalonians 5:18)

"By him therefore let us offer the sacrifice of praise to God continually, that is, the fruit of our lips giving thanks to his name." (Hebrews 13:15)

"The four and twenty elders fall down before him that sat on the throne, and worship him that liveth for ever and ever, and cast their crowns before the throne, saying, Thou art worthy, O Lord, to receive glory and honour and power : for thou hast created all things, and for thy pleasure they are and were created." (Revelation 4:10-11)

"Saying with a loud voice, Fear God, and give glory to him; for the hour of his judgment is come: and worship him that made heaven, and earth, and the sea, and the fountains of waters." (Revelation 14:7)

"And a voice came out of the throne, saying, Praise our God, all ye his servants, and ye that fear him, both small and great." (Revelation 19:5)

The first tongue employed by Satan and used as a weapon against mankind and the work of God was that of the serpent. Satan now a fallen angel, a spiritual being, disguised himself in the serpent's body in order to carry out his diabolical plan against God, and our *first parents*. It was a tongue filled with deceit and lies that forever changed the destiny of mankind as Adam and Eve succumbed to the adversary and ended up losing their home in the Garden of Eden.

The tongue is very powerful, let us therefore seek to use it always as a *servant* and never as a master. In addition to worshipping God with the tongue, let us also seek to use it to encourage others in our daily living. Solomon declared in Proverbs 18:21: **"Death and life are in the power of the tongue: and they that love it shall eat the fruit thereof."** Let us therefore use our tongue to speak beautiful healing words into each others lives instead of cruel negative words that break down lives. We are warned by Jesus in Matthew 12:36-37 that we will be held accountable for every idle word on the day of judgement for by our words we will be justified and by our words we will be condemned. Since we are liable for those words that we speak and will be justified or condemned by those words, it is imperative that we cease using the tongue in an ungodly manner and instead renew the mind and seek to be partakers of the fruit of the Spirit rather than the works of the flesh. Seek to speak words of encouragement in another's life and not words that will hurt and tear down your fellow human being, bless and not curse, build and not tear down—Satan brought death to mankind using the tongue of the serpent, don't allow him to use yours in his continued quest to keep mankind in a state of death. Remember that Christ gave His life on Calvary's cross to give you life anew, choose life today and not death—the choice is yours. Joshua made his choice, he said: **"As for me and my house, we will serve the Lord."** (Joshua 24:15b)

> **"Knowing this, that our old man is crucified with him, that the body of sin might be destroyed, that henceforth we should not serve sin. For he that is dead is freed from sin."** (Romans 6:6-7)

"Submit yourselves therefore to God. Resist the devil, and he will flee from you. Draw nigh to God, and he will draw nigh to you. Cleanse your hands, ye sinners; and purify your hearts, ye double minded"

(James 4:7-8)

The Tongue as a Master

"These six things doth the Lord hate: yea, seven are an abomination unto him: A proud look, a lying tongue, and hands that shed innocent blood, An heart that deviseth wicked imaginations, feet that be swift in running to mischief, A false witness that speaketh lies, and he that soweth discord among brethren." (Proverbs 6:16-19)

The tongue as a master is all-embracing in its assault: Functioning sometimes like a plague—its effect is far-reaching and devastating to those in its path. Other times, it's like a lethal weapon twisting, curling, slithering and stretching as it changes shape to effectively launch its attack. It operates as an arrow, a knife, a sword, an out of control fire, methodically steering the pathway leading to rebellion, and destruction; it wears very ugly labels and when this weapon is drawn it is with intent to maim and devastate—it leaves deep scars, some may take a lifetime to heal. The sins of the tongue are deeply buried in narcissism and are motivated by the works of the flesh that is always seeking to satisfy the lustful appetite of the carnal man. The ungodly tongue has brought down governments and churches, destroyed reputations, ruined careers, wrecked marriages, torn families apart and changed lives forever.

When the tongue is operating as a master it simply means that the flesh has over-powered the spirit and the tongue is now out of control. A tongue out of control is a lethal weapon. It is under the control of Satan, the adversary of mankind from the beginning, whose only objective is to hurt mankind. We should therefore always remember that the tongue becomes a dangerous weapon every time we use it against our fellow human being in an ungodly manner.

God has commanded us to Love others as we love ourselves. When we engage in the sins of the tongue we are not functioning in love and as a result are in direct breach of God's command. In 1 Corinthians 13 we read: **"Though I speak with the tongues of men and of angels, and have not charity, I am become as sounding brass, or a tinkling cymbal...And now abideth faith, hope, charity, these three; but the greatest of these is charity."** Love (charity) is the greatest gift, a multitude is accomplished through love.

As a master the tongue knows no boundary it skips over everything in its path regardless of magnitude or shape—like a forest fire it races furiously out of control until it drains the life from its helpless victim.

"Speak not evil one of another, brethren. He that speaketh evil of his brother, and judgeth his brother, speaketh evil of the law, and judgeth the law: but if thou judge the law, thou art not a doer of the law, but a judge. There is one lawgiver, who is able to save and to destroy: who art thou that judgest another?" (James 4:11-12)

Labels of the Ungodly Tongue:

There are several labels used to describe the ungodly tongue some of which I will discuss in greater detail. They are: Accusing Tongue, Backbiting Tongue, Beguiling Tongue, Belittling Tongue, Betraying Tongue, Boastful Tongue, Complaining Tongue, Compulsive Tongue, Cursing Tongue, Deceitful Tongue, Discouraging Tongue, Divisive Tongue, Doubting Tongue, Gossiping Tongue, Harsh Tongue, Intimidating Tongue, Judgmental Tongue, Manipulative Tongue, Meddling Tongue, Proud Tongue, Rude Tongue, Slandering Tongue, Retaliating Tongue.

Take a good look at some of the arsenal associated with the adversary of mankind, Satan. These missiles are all designed to be self-serving, nevertheless, many among us find them very desirable. They give the impression and the feel of empowerment as we cut down to size those we dislike or those who oppose us. It gives the ultimate 'feel-good' moments, as we plunder and take from society the things we think we need to climb to the pinnacle. I say to you beware of that ungodly tongue you are tempted to use as the ladder that will take you to your desired peak.

Remember always, that the devil is in control of the ungodly tongue for he has his seat deep in the heart attached to that tongue. As the devil showcases the rewards he has laid up for you, bear in mind that the devil's reward is temporary and that there is a consequence for yielding to the devil. Bear in mind also that when you allow yourself to be employed by the devil, you are not only hurting those you touch but you are also hurting yourself—the devil is the only winner; a temporary winner, I might add, for his days of plundering on this earth are getting shorter everyday.

So often we watch as happy homes are wrecked by one or any combination of the evil strongholds listed in this chapter. All of these are by-products of a heart overwhelmed by the works of the flesh. God in His Word commands us to love our neighbour as our self. If we love our neighbour as our self there is no way we would seek to hurt each other and it would be a difficult task for Satan to use us to destroy our fellow man. The Word of God should be a light unto our path dwelling in our hearts always to keep Satan away.

Brief Glance at the Proverbial Ungodly Tongue at Work:

Accusing Tongue:

"Woman, where are those thine accusers? Hath no man condemned thee?" (John 8:10b)

Those who seek to accuse are always filled with flaws of their own and it is not surprising for they are agents of the devil. Satan is a master of accusation—all ungodly tongue and every sinful act originated with Satan. Satan's accusations against those who seek the Lord are not prompted by disapproval of their sins. He gloats in their defective characters for he knows that only through their contravention of God's law can he acquire power over them.

> **"But chiefly them that walk after the flesh in the lust of uncleanness, and despise government. Presumptuous are they, self-willed, they are not afraid to speak evil of dignities. Whereas angels, which are greater in power and might, bring not railing accusation against them before the Lord."**
> (2 Peter 2:10-11)

In the books of Job, Zachariah, and Jude we see Satan directly involved in this type of behaviour. When we first meet Job, we are introduced to him as a man that was perfect and upright, one that feared God and steered clear of evil. Naturally, Satan would not be pleased with Job, this man who hated evil and was a friend of God, and so he laid a trap for Job. He put forth an accusation; in essence, he wanted to see Job wallow in grief, sickness, and poverty for he felt certain that if Job was brought to the level of extensive suffering then Job would blame God and embrace evil and thus sin against God—Satan wanted Job in his own camp. The ever so bold and eloquent Satan showed up before God and dipped in his bag of tricks. He said that Job was only true to God because God was protecting Job and everything that Job possessed. God who sees the heart of all men knew better so He moved His hand of protection from around Job and allowed Satan to have his way with Job's possessions. Job, a true worshipper of God, came out refined as pure gold—proving Satan to be a confounded liar. Satan even employed Job's own wife in the battle against Job: **"Then said his wife unto him, Dost thou still retain thine integrity? curse God, and die. But he said unto her, Thou speakest as one of the foolish women speaketh. What? Shall we receive good at the hand of God, and shall we not receive evil? In all this did not Job sin with his lips."** (Job 2:9-10)

Satan also brought an accusation against Moses, the loyal servant of God. Moses, as documented in Exodus 2:11-15, killed an Egyptian and buried his body in the sand and as a result had to flee from Pharaoh to the land of Midian. When Moses became old and eventually died, he was buried by God, therefore, Satan has no knowledge of his burial place. **"So Moses the servant of the Lord died there in the land of Moab, according to the word of the Lord. And he buried him in a valley in the land of Moab, over against Beth–pe'-or: but no man knoweth of his sepulchre unto this day."** (Deuteronomy 34:5-6) Satan, having knowledge of this event in Egypt when Moses was a young man felt that he was entitled to have Moses' body and so he brought a railing accusation against Moses in his quest to win the case that Moses belonged to him. The archangel, Michael, did not argue with Satan but instead rebuked him. **"Yet Michael the archangel, when contending with the devil he disputed about the body of Moses, durst not bring against him a railing accusation, but said, The Lord rebuke thee."** (Jude 1:9)

Satan even brought an accusation against Joshua. Zechariah, the prophet states:

> **"And he shewed me Joshua the high priest standing before the angel of the Lord, and Satan standing at his right hand to resist him. And the Lord said unto Satan, The Lord rebuke thee, O Satan; even the Lord that hath chosen Jerusalem rebuke thee: is not this a brand plucked out of the fire?"** (Zechariah 3:1-2)

Jesus in dealing with the agents of Satan who had brought before Him a woman they accused of being caught in the act of adultery, made a statement to her accusers: **"He that is without sin among you, let him first cast a stone at her."** (John 8:7b) After making the statement Jesus stooped to write on the ground and when Jesus lifted up His head all her accusers had disappeared silently. Jesus asked the woman, **"Woman, where are those thine accusers? Hath no man condemned thee?"** (John 8:10b)

An accusing tongue is guaranteed to stir up wrath and forge a gap between the accuser and the accused. Let's face it, when we take on the accusing tongue we put the negative energy to work and without a doubt we open the door to discord. Once this door is opened the possibility for emotional upheaval and or outrageous behaviour is endless. Taking on the accusing tongue is never our job. God is the only judge; all judgment should be left to him. Our righteousness is like filthy rags; we are saved only through the grace of God through Jesus Christ. Paul, the apostle, admonished the church in Galatia, **"Brethren, if a man be overtaken in a fault, ye which are spiritual, restore such an one in the spirit of meekness; considering thyself, lest thou also be tempted."** (Galatians 6:1) We live in a world where Satan, the adversary, roams tirelessly seeking whom he may devour. Satan aims to plunder and bring perpetual suffering to mankind and he takes no rest from his attacks. He has purposed within his heart to take as many people as he possibly can to the pit of hell and so we have to be our brother's keeper and not our brother's judge. When one falls along the way it is our duty to help them to get back on the road through the Word of God, prayer, and encouragement instead of using the accusing tongue to alienate them and to bury them in their fault(s). Let us bear one another's burden—through your unconditional love and meekness shown in an act of consideration you could very well be the catalyst in someone's life. You may never know just how you helped to make a positive change in that life but that's not important, you don't have to know, the glory belongs to God. You are only a servant who obeyed your master and by doing so you helped your fellow man back on the road and exalted your master in the process—you played the role of the good servant and you will be rewarded by your master in due season.

Don't take Satan's bait and put yourself in the judgment seat for only God is qualified to judge. God will not share His glory with you—He alone is worthy. He is in heaven and we are on earth—His footstool. Just remember what happened to Herod as documented in Acts 12:20-23 when instead of giving God the glory due unto Him, he took it for himself was eaten alive by the maggots. Satan was thrown out of heaven for the same reason—in his evil conceited heart he saw himself as an authority fit to take the place of God, his Creator.

World War II was instigated by Adolf Hitler, an agent of Satan. He put forward an accusing tongue and passed judgment upon a group of people, and took from them all their possessions—later he took from them, their lives in the most gruesome way. And who were these people— God's chosen people—the very people through whom came Jesus Christ, the Redeemer of the world.

The accusing tongue is one of Satan's sharp weapons. As you might recall when he approached Eve in the Garden of Eden he accosted her with a subtle tone of accusation against God: **"Yea, hath God said, Ye shall not eat of every tree of the garden?"** (Genesis 3:1b) Satan continued the conversation with Eve and assured her that she would not die but would be transformed, becoming as gods. Satan implied that this was something desirable and God only wanted to rob them of that privilege when he told them not to eat the fruit from that particular tree. Eve immediately believed Satan and doubted God, thus she found the fruit desirable and did eat from the tree—Satan had a motive and he successfully used an accusing tongue to secure his objective.

Backbiting Tongue:

Paul lists backbiters among those whom God condemns—**"Backbiters, haters of God, despiteful, proud, boasters, inventors of evil things, disobedient to parents."** (Romans 1:30)

In Numbers chapter 12 there is a major incident where Aaron and Miriam privately engaged in a slanderous conversation (also known as backbiting) in which Moses was the subject. According to their conversation they were not happy that Moses had married an Ethiopian woman, neither were they happy about Moses' position as God's prophet—jealousy had reared its ugly head. **"And they said, Hath the Lord indeed spoken only by Moses? hath he not spoken also by us? And the Lord heard it."** (Numbers 12:2)

God was very displeased with them and he acted very quickly calling all three to come to the tabernacle of the congregation where he spoke to Aaron and Miriam about their behaviour. Moses had to pray for them but God felt that Miriam had to take some degree of accountability for her action. Consequently, Miriam was smitten with leprosy and shut out from the camp for seven days. The entire camp was affected in that they had to remain stationary until Miriam was fit to rejoin the congregation. The only reason she was healed after only seven days is because Moses interceded on her behalf.

David states in Psalm 101:5 **"Whoso privily slandereth his neighbour, him will I cut off: him that hath an high look and a proud heart will not I suffer."** Here David is making it known that he will not be a party to any backbiting conversation—he declares that he will cut off the slanderer. This is the attitude we should all take, for a slanderer cannot pass the poison along if there is nobody to listen. We empower the slanderer when we listen to the gossip and all the garbage they drag into our minds but when we resist them, we shame them into silence and hopefully they will begin to think about their action and reformation.

We are constantly reminded by God's Word to be kind to our fellow man and if we would only obey God instead of the adversary our world would be a better place. **"For all the law is fulfilled in one word, even in this; Thou shalt love thy neighbor as thyself. But if ye bite and devour one another, take heed that ye be not consumed one of another."** (Galatians 5:14, 15)

"The north wind driveth away rain: so doth an angry countenance a backbiting tongue." (Proverbs 25:23) There is a relationship between the attitudes of our hearts and the words that come from our mouths. In the same manner as the wind controls the course and destination of the rain clouds, so the anger in our hearts can control the perception and substance of our speech and even our very countenance.

Further References:

"Where no wood is, there the fire goeth out: so where there is no talebearer, the strife ceaseth. As coals are to burning coals, and wood to fire; so is a contentious man to kindle strife. The words of a talebearer are as wounds, and they go down into the innermost parts of the belly. Burning lips and a wicked heart are like a potsherd covered with silver dross." (Proverbs 26:20-23)

"A froward man soweth strife: and a whisperer separateth chief friends." (Proverbs 16:28)

"He that covereth a transgression seeketh love; but he that repeateth a matter separateth very friends." (Proverbs 17:9)

"And above all things have fervent charity among yourselves: for charity shall cover the multitude of sins." (1 Peter 4:8)

"He that keepeth his mouth keepeth his life: but he that openeth wide his lips shall have destruction." (Proverbs 13:3)

Boastful and Proud Tongue:

"The Lord shall cut off all flattering lips, and the tongue that speaketh proud things: Who have said, With our tongue will we prevail; our lips are our own: who is lord over us?" (Psalm 12:3-4)

"But now ye rejoice in your boastings: all such rejoicing is evil. Therefore to him that knoweth to do good, and doeth it not, to him it is sin."
(James 4:16-17)

Pride is an act of rebelliousness against God. Power, authority, influence, capability, faculty, accuracy—these are all words that are foremost in the vocabulary and subsistence of the proud and boastful. They lead a self-absorbed life using their ego as the very basis on which they build and operate. Blinded by narcissism, they wade deeply into ungodliness believing that they do not need God and they are not accountable to a higher authority—becoming a god unto themselves and to those they consider their inferior. They flaunt their worldly possessions, their talents, and their beauty—finely chiseled bodies, beautiful lips, well-defined nose, the list goes on. They boast of the places their influence and capability have taken them and will yet take them. Riding high on the sea of conceit, they employ every ungodly tongue to serve as conduit throughout their domain and in the 'feel-good' zone at 'power peak': boasting, belittling, compulsive, intimidating, judgmental, manipulative, rude, and harsh tongue. There is no limit to their wickedness; self-reliance is their focal point as they seek to triumph and satisfy their lust by any means regardless of the consequence to others. They are so caught up in their own world that they believe their bodies and talents and everything they possess, belong to them. They operate in the very character of Satan who used the gifts bestowed upon him by God to glorify his vain self and to interfere with God's plans for mankind.

"Boasting is self-centered, it promotes self, and discounts others. Thus, it prevents us from loving because love is a selfless act.

Nebuchadnezzar was a proud and boastful man; the stench of his pride rose up to heaven. In his pride he boasted, **"Is not this great Babylon, that I have built for the house of the kingdom by the might of my power, and for the honour of my majesty?"** (Daniel 4:30b) God had to discipline him immediately; the words had barely left his mouth when his heart was replaced with that of an animal. He took on the characteristics of animals and went out to the pasture to eat grass just like an oxen: **"[H]e was driven from men, and did eat grass as oxen, and his body was wet with the dew of heaven, till his hairs were grown like eagles' feathers, and his nails like birds' claws."** (Daniel 4:33b)

King Nebuchadnezzar got a lesson in humility and he *did* pay attention. These were his words at the end of that unforgettable lesson:

> **"And at the end of the days I Nebuchadnezzar lifted up mine eyes unto heaven, and mine understanding returned unto me, and I blessed the most High, and I praised and honoured him that liveth for ever, whose dominion is an everlasting dominion, and his kingdom is from generation to generation. Now I Nebuchadnezzar praise and extol and honour the King of heaven, all whose works are truth, and his ways judgment: and those that walk in pride he is able to abase."** (Daniel 4: 34, 37)

We need not boast to enhance our sense of worth because everything we possess in terms of physical beauty, talent, and property belongs to God, we are only stewards. Any boasting we do should be boasting in the Lord as He is at work in and through us and our achievements. Paul in his first letter to the Corinthian church said, **"That according as it is written, he that glorieth, let him glory in the Lord."** (1 Corinthians 1:31)

In Psalm 8:3-4 David in communing with God said these words: **"When I consider thy heavens, the work of thy fingers, the moon and the stars, which thou hast ordained; What is man, that thou art mindful of him: and the son of man that thou visitest him?"** James found it necessary to remind us that our life is like a vapor that appears for a little time and then vanishes away.

The Word of God declares:

> **"For the wicked boasteth of his heart's desire, and blesseth the covetous, whom the Lord abhorreth."** (Psalm 10:3)

> **"They that trust in their wealth, and boast themselves in the multitude of their riches; none of them can by any means redeem his brother, nor give to God a ransom for him"** (Psalm 49:6-7)

> **"Whoso boasteth himself of a false gift is like clouds and wind without rain"** (Proverbs 25:14)

"Boast not thyself of tomorrow; for thou knowest not what a day may bring forth" (Proverbs 27:1)

"But now ye rejoice in your boastings: all such rejoicing is evil." (James 4:16)

Complaining Tongue:

In his letter to the Philippians Paul said, **"Do all things without murmurings and disputings: That ye may be blameless and harmless, the sons of God, without rebuke, in the midst of a crooked and perverse nation, among whom ye shine as lights in the world."** (Philippians 2:14-15)

Most people shun complainers because they spew out much bitterness making it depressing and difficult to be around them. The complaining tongue is a conduit for negative energy; it breeds discontentment, festers like a sore, spreads ill-will, lowers morale, weakens leadership, and puts at risk operations that would otherwise have been viable.

Some of us, even Christians, put forward a complaining tongue continually. We complain about the weather, our homes, our children, our jobs, our vehicles, our looks, our talent—the list is never ending. In reality we are saying to God who has promised to supply our needs that He has failed us, we don't trust his judgment. You must never forget that God knows everyone of His children. He knew us before we were formed in the womb. He knows our strengths and weaknesses as well as our maturity. Many of us would like to be in the same job as another earning a higher income but the question is: Would you be able to handle the success that that job brings? We look at many of the Hollywood crowd for several generations—success became a curse rather than a blessing. There are so many who have lost themselves in alcohol and drugs and lewd lifestyles and never really find happiness. When the children of Israel entered the Promised Land, God did not allow them to take all the land at once. He waited for their number to increase for without enough people to inhabit the land the wild animals would have occupied and this would be a threat to their safety.

Paul the Apostle said,

> **"Not that I speak in respect of want: for I have learned, in whatsoever state I am, therewith to be content. I know both how to be abased, and I know how to abound: every where and in all things I am instructed both to be full and to be hungry, both to abound and to suffer need. I can do all things through Christ which strengtheneth me."** (Philippians 4:11-13)

The story is told of a man who was always complaining about not having a pair of shoes to wear. Then, one day he saw a man without feet. It struck him that he was in a better position than this man who had no feet to walk. For the first time, he realized how blessed he was and from that day forward he stopped complaining about having no shoes to wear. It is so easy to complain about the things we don't have or can't have now, rather than to give thanks for what we do have. The children of Israel displayed this same type of behavior during their journey in the wilderness.

Although the Lord God had demonstrated his loving care for them by bringing them out from harsh bondage in Egypt, and feeding them with manna from heaven during their journey in the wilderness, they remained a thankless, unholy, and complaining people. The Lord was not pleased with them and they did suffer the consequences. Their complaining meant that they were not satisfied with the provision God had made for them. They showed ungratefulness and lack of trust in God the Almighty even after the many wonders He performed in their presence.

"How long shall I bear with this evil congregation, which murmur against me? I have heard the murmurings of the children of Israel, which they murmur against me. Say unto them, As truly as I live, saith the Lord, as ye have spoken in mine ears, so will I do to

you: Your carcases will fall in this wilderness; and all that were numbered of you, according to your whole number, from twenty years old and upward, which have murmured against me." (Numbers 14:27-29)

As parents, we expect our children to be satisfied with what we provide for them and we expect them to accept and trust us in the decisions we make on their behalf but by the same token we do not show our Father, the Almighty God, the same respect. Who are we to take such attitude? Just remember, we are a created being. In Matthew 7:9-11 Jesus said: **"Or what man is there of you, whom if his son ask bread, will he give him a stone? Or if he ask a fish, will he give him a serpent? If he then, being evil, know how to give good gifts unto your children, how much more shall your Father which is in heaven give good things to them that ask him?"**

Christ is our example. He was nailed to the cross but he did not complain. **"He was oppressed, and he was afflicted, yet he opened not his mouth: he is brought as a lamb to the slaughter, and as a sheep before her shearers is dumb, so he openeth not his mouth."** (Isaiah 53:7)

When the children of Israel became dissatisfied with being ruled by judges they went to Samuel and demanded a king to rule over them. Samuel felt rejected but God told him that he was not the one being rejected—the children of Israel had rejected God as their King. Israel was presumptuous in asking for a king and that rejection of God was the rudiment for the later sorrows of the Chosen People. Their punishment was in getting what they asked for. They could have saved themselves much suffering and pain had they remained satisfied with what God had chosen for them.

We should not take on the complaining tongue. It suggests that we are not satisfied with what God has given us. God is the father, he is the creator, the world and everything therein belongs to him. He is the father who provides for us his children, the just and the unjust. We must never forget that God knows our beginning and our end. Lucifer changed his destiny and that of mankind when he decided that he wanted to be what he was not created to be. Let us seek the perfect will of God in our lives and not His permissive will.

Cursing Tongue:

"Their throat is an open sepulchre; with their tongues they have used deceit; the poison of asps is under their lips: whose mouth is full of cursing and bitterness"
(Romans 3:13-14)

Balak, the Moabite king was greatly afraid when he saw the Israelites camped on the plains of Moab, east of Jordan. He was aware that they had conquered the Amorites and had taken their land and he realized that his country could be the next target. He wasted no time in sending for a man called Balaam to curse the Israelites. Balaam's work was held in high esteem in that idolatrous nation of Moab and it was reputed that he whom Balaam blessed was blessed, and he whom Balaam cursed was cursed—King Balak got himself the best man in the land for the job but the best was not good enough. God instructed Balaam not to curse these people because they are blessed but Balaam put himself in a compromising position and would have been killed by an angel had not the ass on which he was riding miraculously spoke to him. In the end, Balaam and Balak went to three different locations to pronounce curse upon the children of Israel but each time Balaam opened his mouth he pronounced a blessing instead of a curse.

> **"And he took up his parable, and said Rise up, Balak, and hear; hearken unto me, thou son of Zippor: God is not a man, that he should lie; neither the son of man, that he should repent: hath he said, and shall he not do it? Or hath he spoken, and shall he not make it good? Behold, I have received commandment to bless: and he hath blessed; and I cannot reverse it."** (Numbers 23:18-20)

God further used Balaam to prophesy over the Children of Israel: "**Blessed is he that blesseth thee, and cursed is he that curseth thee.**" (Numbers 24:9b)

"**As he loved cursing, so let it come unto him: as he delighted not in blessing, so let it be far from him. As he clothed himself with cursing like as with his garment, so let it come into his bowels like water, and like oil into his bones.**" (Psalm 109:17-18) Many people curse because their life is unhappy; they make this unhappiness known with their debauched speech as the heart overflows with all sorts of damaging emotions. This text shows that we are kept unhappy because of the bad choices we make. Clearly we cannot expect to have blessing in our lives if all we do is curse others. We have got to be prepared to reap what we sow—we cannot reap blessing if we sow cursing.

> "**Finally, be ye all of one mind, having compassion one of another, love as brethren, be pitiful, be courteous: Not rendering evil for evil, or railing for railing: but contrariwise blessing; knowing that ye are thereunto called, that ye should inherit a blessing. For he that will love life, and see good days, let him refrain his tongue from evil, and his lips that they speak no guile.**" (1 Peter 3:8-10)

Discouraging and DoubtingTongue:

Moses was directed by God to go in and possess the land but when he gave command according to the directions from the Lord, the Children of Israel put forth the doubting tongue and instead of going in to conquer the land they requested of Moses that some of their men be sent in, to search out the land first. Moses gave in to them sending twelve spies, one from each tribe, to secretly go into the Promised Land to check it out.

> **"Behold, the Lord thy God hath set the land before thee: go up and possess it, as the Lord God of thy fathers had said unto thee; fear not, neither be discouraged. And he came near unto me every one of you, and said, We will send men before us, and they shall search us out the land, and bring us word again by what way we must go up, and into what cities we shall come".** (Deuteronomy 1:21-22)

Moses faced rebellion in the wilderness after 11 of these spies came back with bad report. The negative report they brought back greatly discouraged the people to the extent that they murmured against the Lord complaining that the Lord hated them and had brought them up out of Egypt to deliver them into the hand of the Amorites to destroy them. So great was the anger of God against them that He did not allow any of that generation, except for

Caleb who had brought back a good report, to enter the Promised Land. They wandered around in the wilderness for 40 years until that generation died and their children, a new generation, rose up to take their places—the new generation entered the Promised Land. Their doubting and discouraging tongue also caused Moses to die before reaching the Promised Land.

> **"Surely there shall not one of these men of this evil generation see that good land, which I sware to give unto your fathers, Save Caleb the son of Jephunneh; he shall see it, and to him will I give the land that he hath trodden upon, and to his children, because he hath wholly followed the Lord. Also the Lord was angry with me for your sakes, saying, Thou also shalt not go in thither. But Joshua the son of Nun, which standeth before thee, he shall go in thither: encourage him: for he shall cause Israel to inherit it."**
> (Deuteronomy 1:35-38)

In Luke chapter 1 we meet Zacharias, a priest, a man adept in all the wonders that God had done in the lives of his descendants, the Israelites and that of their father Abraham, and Sarah who had given birth to Isaac in old age. Zacharias had been given the good news that God had answered his prayers and that his wife Elisabeth would conceive and bear a son, but instead of welcoming the news with praise and thanksgiving he listened to the lying words Satan had put in his thoughts and put forward a doubting tongue. Zacharias put into words the reasoning of his carnal thoughts as to why the promise of God delivered by the angel Gabriel was impossible. God immediately silenced that doubting tongue and only loosened it after the child was born and brought in for circumcision on the eighth day. The moment Zacharias wrote the baby's name as given to him by the angel Gabriel, in the temple on that fateful day, his speech was restored. Zacharias had learned a very important lesson. Once his tongue was loosened he started praising God and he became filled with the Holy Ghost and started to prophesy. A doubting tongue can unwittingly spew out words of hindrance and destruction putting up roadblocks in a pathway that had been previously freed from all obstacles. **"Death and life are in the power of the tongue"**—very powerful words they are and we owe it to ourselves to pay attention to them—recorded in Proverbs 18:21a.

During Jesus' ministry on earth he could not perform many miracles in His hometown, Nazareth, because of the doubters there. The unbelief in Nazareth interfered with Jesus' work. Mark 6:1-2, 5-6 states:

> **"And he went out from thence, and came into his own country; and his disciples**

> follow him. And when the Sabbath day was
> come, he began to teach in the synagogue:
> and many hearing him were astonished,
> saying, From whence hath this man these
> things? and what wisdom is this which is
> given unto him, that even such mighty
> works are wrought by his hands? And he
> could there do no mighty work, save that
> he laid his hands upon a few sick folk, and
> healed them. And he marveled because of
> their unbelief. And he went round about the
> villages, teaching."

Jesus appeared to his disciples after his resurrection but at the time Thomas, one of His disciples, was absent. When the others told Thomas about the appearance he did not believe—"**The other disciples therefore said unto him, We have seen the Lord. But he said unto them, Except I shall see in his hands the print of the nails, and put my finger into the print of the nails, and thrust my hand into his side, I will not believe.**" (John 20:25)

Eight days later all the disciples were together and again Jesus appeared to them and spoke directly with the doubtful Thomas.

> "Then saith he to Thomas, Reach hither thy
> finger and behold my hands; and reach hither
> thy hand, and thrust it into my side: and be

**not faithless, but believing. And Thomas
answered and said unto him, My Lord and
my God. Jesus saith unto him, Thomas,
because thou hast seen me, thou hast
believed: blessed are they that have not seen,
and yet have believed."** (John 20:27-29)

John Mark, the author of the gospel of Mark, then a
young man, went with Paul and Barnabas on their first
missionary journey but did not perform satisfactorily and
eventually deserted them at Pamphylia. It is clear that
Paul did not appreciate John Mark's action and so when
he and Barnabas decided to go on the second missionary
journey and Barnabas wanted to take John Mark along
Paul completely objected to this. Paul felt that it was not
good to take John Mark along because of his past behavior
on the first missionary journey. Barnabas, however, was
determined to give John Mark another chance regardless
of what Paul thought, and so rather than leaving the young
John Mark behind he chose not to travel with Paul. In Acts
15:39 we read of the intensity of that dissention: **"And
the contention was so sharp between them, that they
departed asunder one from the other: and so Barnabas
took Mark, and sailed unto Cyprus;"** Barnabas realized
that this young man had erred but he was not willing to
push him aside, he felt that he should be given another
chance. Barnabas was by all account a humble man who

possessed the heart of a servant. He saw the good in others and because of this attitude there was much growth in the early church. This is a commendable quality that we could all nurture in our lives today for it would certainly enhance our impact as Christians. I am sure that John Mark appreciated the opportunity for he did get his act together and went on to write the book of Mark.

Paul should not have been astonished that Barnabas stood up to him about taking John Mark along on the journey. Ironically, Barnabas spoke up for Paul when as a young convert he was still under a cloud of suspicion and now we see him standing up for John Mark when Paul had given up on him. Acts 9:26-27 declares:

> **"And when Saul was come to Jerusalem, he assayed to join himself to the disciples: but they were all afraid of him, and believed not that he was a disciple. But Barnabas took him, and brought him to the apostles, and declared unto them how he had seen the Lord in the way, and that he had spoken to him, and how he had preached boldly at Damascus in the name of Jesus."**

Barnabas, the Son of Encouragement, stood alongside Paul when everyone else shunned the new convert once known for grave atrocities among the early Christian community. It is interesting to note that later on in his ministry Paul saw the fruit of Barnabas' work in the life of the young John Mark—Paul wrote in 2 Timothy 4:9-11: **"Do thy diligence to come shortly unto me: For Demas hath forsaken me, having loved this present world, and is departed unto Thessalonica; Crescens to Galatia, Titus unto Dalmatia. Only Luke is with me. Take Mark, and bring him with thee: for he is profitable to me for the ministry."**

Had Barnabas discouraged John Mark his life could have taken a negative turn. A word of encouragement means much to a soul cast down and discouraged, a soul who constantly struggles to stay on the right path—encouragement strengthens while discouragement destroys. David was a man who was able to encourage himself in the Lord in his deepest moment of despair: **"And David was greatly distressed; for the people spake of stoning him, because the soul of all the people was grieved, every man for his sons and for his daughters: but David encouraged himself in the Lord his God."** (1 Samuel 30:6)

Not many are strong enough to operate as David did so we should always seek to encourage those who are overwhelmed by their particular situation.

Lying Tongue:

A lying tongue comes from a lying heart. Lies, deceit, slander, and pride, started in the heart of Satan and caused his demise. A lying tongue formulates mischief and works deceitfully. **"Thy tongue deviseth mischiefs; like a sharp razor, working deceitfully. Thou lovest evil more than good; and lying rather than to speak righteousness. Thou lovest all devouring words, O thou deceitful tongue."** (Psalm 52:2-4)

The Day of Pentecost was a time of new beginning for mankind—Christ had been crucified and had arose from the dead, and ascended into heaven and the comforter he had promised his disciples had come to earth. Five thousand souls were saved on that day and many were added to the church daily. The newly formed church was of one accord they were conscious of each others needs and those who had possessions sold it voluntarily and brought the money to Peter to be used accordingly. The old serpent was not far away, he entered the heart of new converts Ananias and his wife, Sapphira. They went out and sold their house but conspired between themselves to lie about the amount they had sold the property for. When Ananias brought the money to Peter he was asked if that was what he had sold the house for and he answered in the affirmative. Peter knew that he was lying and spoke to him sternly: **"Ananias, why hath Satan filled thine heart to lie to the Holy Ghost, and to keep back part of the price of the land?"** (Acts 5:3) Peter told Ananias that he had lied to God—his lie cost him his life. His wife Sapphira came in three hours after her husband was dead and told the same lie as her husband and she also fell to the floor and died. This couple allowed Satan to use their tongue as an instrument of lies and in the process they lost their lives.

The Lord hates a lying tongue. Throughout the Bible we are reminded of this. In John 8:44 Jesus declared: **"Ye are of your father the devil, and the lusts of your father ye will do. He was a murderer from the beginning, and abode not in the truth, because there is no truth in him. When he speaketh a lie, he speaketh of his own: for he is a liar, and the father of it."**

The psalmist declares in Psalm 120:2, **"Deliver my soul, O Lord, from lying lips, and from a deceitful tongue."**

Again, the Bible states in Proverbs 12:13 & 19 **"The wicked is snared by the transgression of his lips: but the just shall come out of trouble. "The lip of truth shall be established for ever: but a lying tongue is but for a moment."**

As well, Revelation 21:8 states: **"But the fearful, and unbelieving, and the abominable, and murderers, and whoremongers, and sorcerers, and idolaters, and all liars, shall have their part in the lake which burneth with fire and brimstone which is the second death."**

"Wherefore putting away lying, speak every man truth with his neighbour: for we are members one of another. . . . Let no corrupt communication proceed out of your mouth, but that which is good to the use of edifying, that it may minister grace unto the hearers. . . . Let all bitterness, and wrath, and anger, and clamour, and evil speaking, be put away from you, with all malice:"

Ephesians 4:25, 29, 31

Bringing the Evil Tongue into Captivity

"But I say unto you, That every idle word that men shall speak, they shall give account thereof in the day of judgment. For by thy words thou shalt be justified, and by thy words thou shalt be condemned."
(Matthew 12:36-37)

"Let no corrupt communications proceed out of your mouth, but that which is good to the use of edifying that it may minister grace unto the hearers. And grieve not the Holy Spirit of God, whereby ye are sealed unto the day of redemption. Let all bitterness, and wrath, and anger, and clamour, and evil speaking, be put away from you, with all malice: And be ye kind one to another, tenderhearted, forgiving one another, even as God for Christ's sake hath forgiven you."
(Ephesians 4:29-32)

The sins of the tongue have their roots buried deeply in ungodliness and wrapped in the work of the flesh and are always self-serving. There has been a continuous war between the spirit and the flesh, and the tongue has proved to be a very effective weapon in Satan's camp. The tongue can, however, be brought into captivity when we choose to abandon the sinful nature with which we were born and walk in newness of life replacing the old self with the spirit of God who indwells us and guides us when we accept Jesus Christ as our personal savior.

God has created us and has given us free will to choose where we will spend eternity. While God is pleased and there is great rejoicing in heaven over one sinner that repents God will not force us to spend eternity with Him—it has to be an independent choice and must be made during our lifetime. The choice we make will determine whether we spend eternity in the presence of God surrounded by His love, joy, peace, and light or whether we will be separated from Him and cast in outer darkness. It is an ultimate choice; there is no middle ground because God is holy. He is the light and He is love—the absolute opposite to ungodliness, and darkness. Salvation determines our eternal destiny and is therefore the most important decision we will ever make in our lives.

As we take on the walk with Christ yielding ourselves to Him daily in thought and willingness to obey and ask

God to work in us, He will continue His marvellous work of stabilizing our thoughts according to His thoughts. We will grow and mature spiritually as we read His Word daily and seek Him through fasting and prayer. You will begin to notice that even in the sub-conscious your heart is always in the act of worship, there maybe a song of rejoicing or praise or the Word of God bubbling in your heart. As you continue to water your heart with the Word of God you will find you have no desire for the sins of the tongue or any type of sinfulness for that matter—your desire will be to worship God continually and to please Him in your daily living.

> **"Thy word have I hid in my heart, that I might not sing against thee"** (Psalm 119:11)

> **"Let the words of my mouth, and the meditation of my heart, be acceptable in thy sight, O Lord, my strength, and my redeemer."** (Psalm 19:14)

> **"And they that are Christ's have crucified the flesh with the affections and lusts."** (Galatians 5:24)

> **"And he said to them all, If any man will come after me, let him deny himself, and take up his cross daily, and follow me. For**

> **whosoever will save his life shall lose it: but whosoever will lose his life for my sake, the same shall save it."** (Luke 9:23-24)

> **"Neither yield ye your members as instruments of unrighteousness unto sin: but yield yourselves unto God, as those that are alive from the dead, and your members as instruments of righteousness unto God."** (Romans 6:13)

It is important that we as followers of Christ spend time in prayer and in His Word on a daily basis for Satan is always watching for the opportunity to return to his old house and he will come in by way of the weakest area. Don't forget, he is familiar with our weaknesses and he is determined to take as many people as he can to that place of torment that has been prepared for him.

Always remember that God is a God of mercy and love and He has built a new road to take us back to Him but He will not force us to take that road or to stay on that road against our will. We can, however, depend on Him to give us covering if we stay in close communication with Him during the journey along this new road.

> **"Finally, my brethren, be strong in the Lord, and in the power of his might. Put on the whole armour of God, that ye may**

be able to stand against the wiles of the devil. For we wrestle not against flesh and blood, but against principalities, against powers, against the rulers of the darkness of this world, against spiritual wickedness in high places. Wherefore take unto you the whole armour of God, that ye may be able to withstand in the evil day, and having done all, to stand. Stand therefore, having your loins girt about with truth, and having on the breastplate of righteousness; And your feet shod with the preparation of the gospel of peace; Above all, taking the shield of faith, wherewith ye shall be able to quench all the fiery darts of the wicked. And take the helmet of salvation, and the sword of the Spirit, which is the word of God: Praying always with all prayer and supplication in the Spirit, and watching thereunto with all perseverance and supplication for all saints; And for me, that utterance may be given unto me, that I may open my mouth boldly, to make known the mystery of the gospel, For which I am an ambassador in bonds: that therein I may speak boldly, as I ought to speak." (Ephesians 6:10-20)

When we worship the Lord we not only honor and magnify Him but we ourselves are strengthened and edified—taking on the character of God. As we continue to worship God in fullness, we will be inclined to embrace His values and gradually take on His characteristics and qualities, although not to His level. Philippians 2:5 declares, **"Let this mind be in you, which was also in Christ Jesus:"** The question is often asked, How do we take on the mind of Christ? Romans 12:2 affirms, **"And be not conformed to this world: but be ye transformed by the renewing of your mind, that ye may prove what is that good, and acceptable, and perfect, will of God."** We renew our minds as we study and meditate on God's Word and worship Him in songs, praises, and by our testimonies. We develop such traits as forgiveness, tenderness, justice, righteousness, purity, kindness, and love. All of this is preparing us for eternal life in heaven with God. We are told in Colossians 3:2: **"Set your affection on things above, not on things on the earth."**

The fruit of the spirit is the divine nature of God and our evidence of perfection. We read in 2 Peter 1: 3, 4, 9:

> **"According as his divine power hath given unto us all things that pertain unto life and godliness, through the knowledge of him that hath called us to glory and virtue: Whereby are given unto us exceeding great**

and precious promises: that by these ye might be partakers of the divine nature, having escaped the corruption that is in the world through lust. But he that lacketh these things is blind, and cannot see afar off, and hath forgotten that he was purged from his old sins."

Ephesians 5: 9-11 tells us: "For the fruit of the Spirit is in all goodness and righteousness and truth; Proving what is acceptable unto the Lord. And have no fellowship with the unfruitful works of darkness, but rather reprove them."

We read in Joshua 24:15: "And if it seem evil unto you to serve the Lord, choose you this day whom ye will serve; whether the gods which your fathers served that were on the other side of the flood, or the gods of the Amorites, in whose land ye dwell: but as for me and my house, we will serve the Lord."

As well Romans 8:6-9 tells us:

"For to be carnally minded is death; but to be spiritually minded is life and peace. Because the carnal mind is enmity against God: for it is not subject to the law of God, neither indeed can be. So then they that are in the flesh cannot please God. But ye are not in the flesh, but in the Spirit, if so be that the Spirit of God dwell in you. Now if any man have not the spirit of Christ, he is none of his."

Romans 8:1 states: "There is therefore now no condemnation to them which are in Christ Jesus, who walk not after the flesh, but after the Spirit."

And finally, we read in Deuteronomy 30:19-20a, "I call heaven and earth to record this day against you, that I have set before you life and death, blessing and cursing: therefore choose life, that both thou and thy seed may live: That thou mayest love the Lord thy God, and that thou mayest obey his voice, and that thou mayest cleave unto him: for he is thy life, and the length of thy days:"

What will you choose? A Spirit-filled existence and life **or** a flesh-driven existence and death?

"Blessed are they that do His Commandments, that they may have right to the tree of life, and may enter in through the gates into the city. For without are dogs, and sorcerers, and whoremongers, and murderers, and idolaters, and whosoever loveth and maketh a lie."

(Revelation 22:14-15)

Helpful References
for Daily Living

"Study to shew thyself approved unto God, a workman that needeth

not to be ashamed, rightly dividing the word of truth"

(2 Timothy 2:15)

Job 5:21	*Psalm 100*
Psalm 5:9	*Psalm 103*
Psalm 12:3-4	*Psalm 109:2*
Psalm 15:1-3	*Psalm 119:172*
Psalm 19:14	*Psalm 120: 3*
Psalm 34:13	*Psalm 149*
Psalm 37:30	*Proverbs 6:2,17*
Psalm 39:1, 3	*Proverbs 10:11,19, 31*
Psalm 64:3	*Proverbs12:18*
Psalm 66:17	*Proverbs15:4*
Psalm 71:24	*Proverbs16:24*
Psalm 73:9	*Proverbs 17:4, 20*

Proverbs 18:21

Proverbs 20:15

Proverbs 21:23

Proverbs 25:11,15, 23

Ecclesiastes 5:6

Ecclesiastes 10:14

Matthew 12:34-37

Colossians 4:6

Romans 3:4,13-14

1 Corinthians 2:1-4

2 Corinthians 12:20

Galatians 6:7-9

Ephesians 4:22-31

Ephesians 5:4

Hebrews 10:24-25

James 1:26

Romans 10:9-10

Romans 6:12-13

James 3:1-12

1 Peter 3:10

Jude 1

"He that overcometh shall inherit all things; and I will be his God, and he shall be my son." (Revelation 21:7)

Reflections

When next you are tempted to use your tongue as a weapon against your fellow human, reflect on these things:

Your unanswered prayers could be a result of the sins of the tongue in your life **"If I regard iniquity in my heart, the Lord will not hear me."** (Psalm 66:18)

~*~

O criticizing tongue
Before you attack
Remember, the roles could have been reversed.
Don't criticize another's looks
Who made you?
The same one who made you made the other
When you criticize another it's Him you criticize
He could have given the other your looks
But He did not, He knows the parcel
that's just right for everyone
he has a purpose for every package
You are fearfully and wonderfully made
Never forget...

~*~

Slandering Tongue

Oh slandering tongue, where will you go today?
Restlessly you twitch, as you carefully select your next victim
Like a graceful butterfly you flutter from desk to desk
Your concern for everyone in your path
deceitfully exudes utter kindness
As you flit with charm.
Oh slanderous tongue how charmingly you conceal such poison
Intent on destroying the prey so carefully chosen.

Unknown to your prey your technique is perfect
You've taken hold of vital information
Your poisonous fang you now sink in
And away you go flying high as a kite

Slanderous tongue I watched you
As you strategically inject the poison all over the city block
Your contagious poison flows swiftly as it vehemently
Drags your victim into utter shame and disgust.

Oh slanderous tongue you refused to be still
Oh slanderous tongue stop! Stop!
You have destroyed another life
Release your fang, you tortuous enemy!

~*~

Life is a journey

On your way you will meet many
Some you will like and others you'll be tempted to dislike
Regardless of your station or position
Treat each with kindness and show your love
For you will pass this way but once

~*~

My Body God's Temple

Don't brag about your good looks or your finely chisled body
It is not yours to keep, it is a gift from God
Carved from the dust of the earth
Meant to house the spirit that lives deep within

You had no say in how you were carved
Accept with joy the body given to you
Keep it clean, never contaminate the spirit residing there
Some day the spirit will fly away
and to the earth your body will return

Trust not in your beauty, flaunt not your beauty
for one day it will surely slip silently away
That elderly man, that elderly woman sitting next to you
gray stringy hair, bent over, emaciated skin
was once young and vibrant just like you.

Spend your time beautifying the inner man
Housed within that case we call the body
For your inner man will never die
He will live through the ages
a place of comfort... or torment.

For by Him were all things created, that are in heaven, and that are in the earth, visible and invisible, whether they be thrones, or dominions, or principalities, or powers: all things were created by Him, and for Him: (Colossians 1:16)

Works Cited

"Discovery of 'hot pepper' receptor in heart may explain chest pain, lead to new treatments" (1 September 2003), online: *Innovations Reports (Forum for Science, Industry and Business)* <http://www.innovations-report.com/html/reports/life_sciences/report-20963.html>.

Kaptchuk, Ted J. <u>The Web That Has No Weaver</u>. Chicago: Contemporary, 2000.

"Opens onto the tongue", online:
Traditional Chinese Medicine and Acupuncture Health Information Organization <http://tcm.health-info.org/Zang%20Fu%20foundation/heart.htm>.

The Holy Bible, King James Version. Nashville: Thomas Nelson, 1976.

Zahner, Matthew R., De-Pei Li, and Shao-Rui Chen, "Hot pepper chemical links tongue to heart" (2 September 2003), online: Penn State Live <http://live.psu.edu/story/3909>.